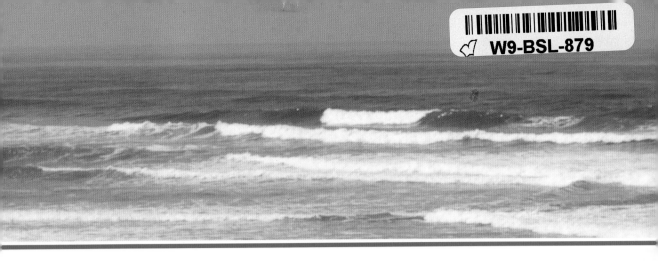

Ultrafit!

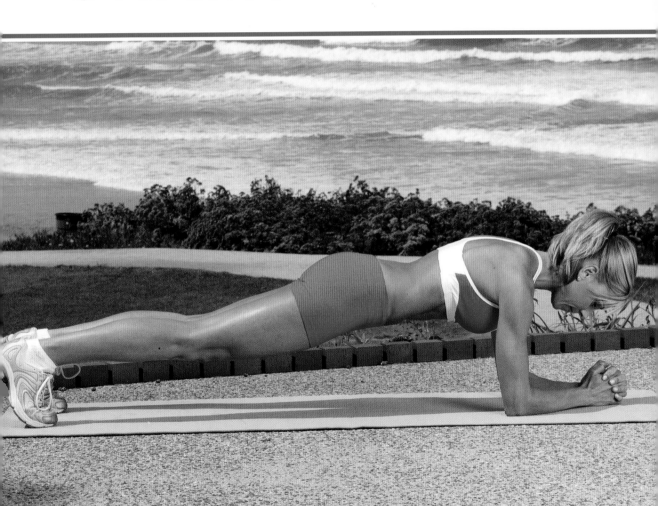

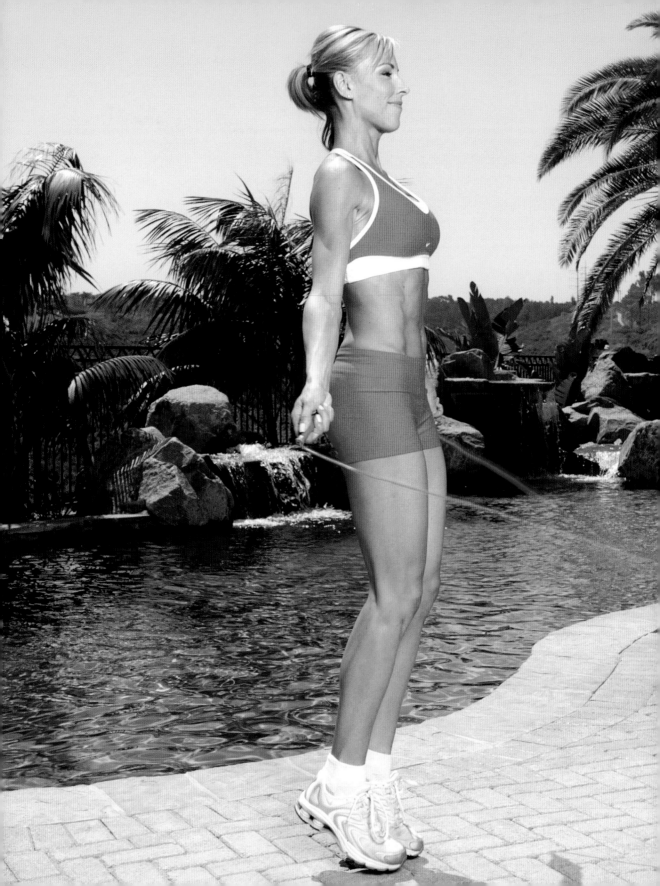

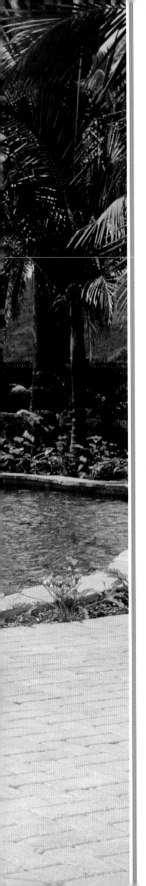

Ultrafit!

Challenging Workouts—Amazing Results

Cindy Whitmarsh

FAIR WINDS

PRESS

GLOUCESTER, MASSACHUSETTS

dedication

To my husband Mike and my babies Jaden and Kendall,
for letting me pursue my dreams. I love you all!

Text © 2006 by Cindy Whitmarsh

First published in the USA in 2006 by
Fair Winds Press, a member of
Quayside Publishing Group
33 Commercial Street
Gloucester, MA 01930

10 09 08 07 06   1 2 3 4 5

ISBN 1-59233-175-0
Library of Congress Cataloging-in-Publication Data

Whitmarsh, Cindy.
  Ultrafit! : challenging workouts-amazing results / Cindy Whitmarsh.
      p. cm.
  Summary: "Workout routines and fitness exersizes to be done at
home"--Provided by publisher.
  Includes bibliographical references and index.
  ISBN 1-59233-175-0
  1. Exercise. 2. Physical fitness. I. Title.
  GV481.W485 2006
  613.7'1--dc22

                             2005024251
Cover design by Howard Grossman/12E Design
Book design by Yee Design
Photography by Allan Penn

Printed and bound in China

The information in this book is for educational purposes only. It is not intended to
replace the advice of a physician or medical practitioner. Please see your health
care provider before beginning any new health program.

what people are saying about **ultra**fit

"I met Cindy Whitmarsh after I had some surgery and needed to make a lifestyle change in my nutrition and fitness levels. I am a military wife and mom of three kids, one of whom has cerebral palsy. Cindy's Ultrafit program showed me it is possible to be a busy, on-the-go mom, and still work out, eat right, and take care of myself. The program is easy to follow and took my likes and dislikes into consideration. It took me to the next level of fitness which allowed me to have the energy to take care of my family. I went from a size 10 to a size 4 and lost 5 percent of my body fat in only 9 weeks!"

—Lori Brown, mother of three, Oceanside, California

"I have been a fitness enthusiast my whole life but I never achieved the lean body definition that I have from the Ultrafit workouts! I learned the benefits of cross training and the importance of core and flexibility training. My wife Kristin and I are nurse practitioners and we recommend the Ultrafit programs to all our clients. Ultrafit is a way of life at our house thanks to Cindy!"

—Kevin Chaussee, Family Nurse Practitioner, Bismarck, North Dakota

"I tried all my life to get leaner. My upper body was always thin but my lower body wasn't. I went through stages 2 and 3 and in 12 weeks I have achieved the lean figure that I have always desired! Cindy's program taught me how to strength train, core train, and interval train! I have so much energy for my two very active boys and my I will follow Ultrafit forever!"

—Cindy Braun, mother of two, San Diego, California

"I did the Ultrafit program in the beginning to prove Cindy wrong. I told her that no exercise or diet had ever worked for me, and she challenged me to try her program. Well, boy, was I wrong! I had results even the first week of the program, and that sparked a small bit of confidence not only in me but also in her program. I now have self-confidence I never had before. I can wear any clothes I want! I never cry when I look in the mirror anymore; I am positive and strong and have the energy to move mountains! My husband says I am now the happy person I was when we got married. That means more to me than anything. I was so inspired by my results and the Ultrafit program that I have now dedicated my life to helping others as well."

—Trish Vasper, Ultrafit Consultant, Frogs Club One, Solana Beach, California

contents

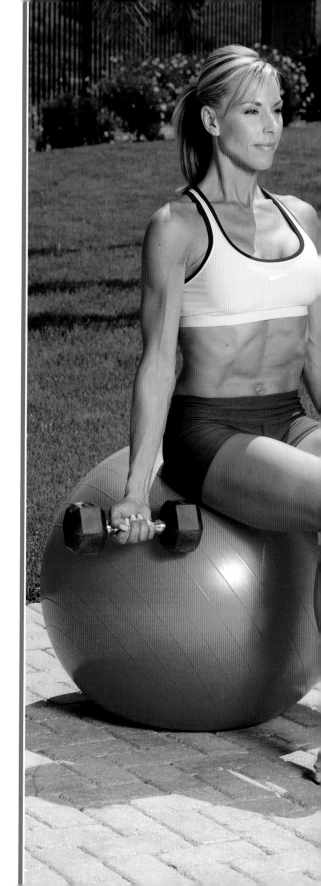

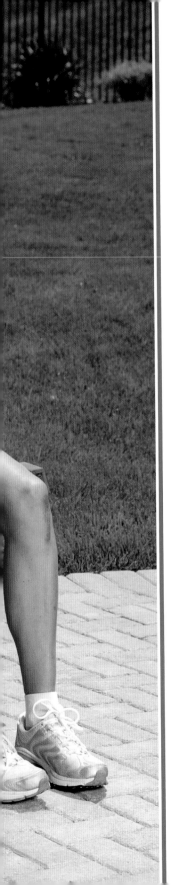

foreword

I met Cindy back in the days when I used to travel to North Dakota and other parts of the world to teach training workshops to other instructors. I have seen her develop into a first-class fitness instructor, trainer, and now entrepreneur. Watching clients go through the 6-week Ultrafit Challenge with Cindy is like watching "Extreme Makeover" without the surgeries. Her clients walk away with their heads high and their shoulders back, proud to show off their well-toned bodies.

Ultrafit is a workout program like no other. If you are tired of the same old workout, or haven't seen changes in your body after years of training then you need this book.

Based on her own experiences and extensive education in the field of health, nutrition, and exercise, Cindy Whitmarsh has designed the ultimate fitness program for both men and women. Whether you are at an early stage of training or an experienced exerciser, you can take your body to the next level with Cindy's personally designed workouts and nutritional programs that have gotten her the body everyone wants! There are no gimmicks, no get-fit-quick mentality or promises she can't keep. Cindy is the real deal and has the body and knowledge to prove it.

Now, read on and let Cindy help you get into the best shape of your life!

Here's to lifelong health and fitness!

Tamilee Webb M.A.
Ms. Buns of Steel
www.webbworkout.com

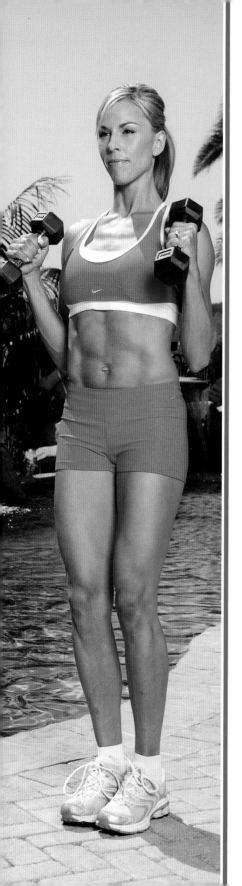

introduction

THE BEGINNINGS OF ULTRAFIT

Being forty pounds overweight is no way to get work as a personal trainer. When I look back now on the way my body was in 1994, I'm amazed that I was able to hold a decent client base. Fresh out of college with a degree in science from North Dakota State University and a background in fitness and nutrition, I had the makings of a great personal trainer and fitness instructor—I had the knowledge, the desire, and the outgoing personality, but I didn't have the body to match my career in guiding people towards better health. The shape I was in made it increasingly difficult to get clients, as my body wasn't one to be admired or envied. I certainly didn't look like I had the sense of self-control I was constantly preaching to my clients! Finally I got to the point where my weight was holding me back for the life I wanted.

It began with my own personal obsession with my weight. I was constantly looking in the mirror and not liking what I was seeing, and even began wearing a sweatshirt wrapped around my rear end while teaching aerobics classes—not the best way to make it look any smaller! One day, I overheard a new member requesting information on personal training at the front desk. I was tempted to approach her and introduce myself, until I heard her say, "I want to meet with a trainer, but not that fat girl trainer you have." Hearing that knocked the air right out of me. At that moment, I came out of my deep abyss of denial and realized that I wasn't the only one who noticed my weight issue. I didn't think I could feel lower, but that same day, I overheard a gentleman on the training floor tell his buddy that I shouldn't be allowed to wear shorts due to the excess cellulite on my legs. I felt shattered, but I was determined to overcome my obesity.

So that was it. That was the day I devoted myself to turning my body around. I rushed home and immediately began designing a plan that would turn my weight problem around, and I knew it would require a total lifestyle change. It meant going cold turkey on the sugar, diet soda, caffeine, and alcohol I had been so hooked on since college. And nutrition was just the beginning—it also meant holding fast to a whole new combination of challenging workouts. What I ultimately developed was the Ultrafit Program, which you now have the opportunity to read about it in this book. I devoted myself to the Ultrafit Program for five months, and I lost those 40 pounds safely and effectively. More importantly, I kept them off. How did I stay motivated? Each week I saw little changes in my body and the way I felt about myself started to improve, along with my self-confidence. The benefits were too great to even consider giving up!

Five months after starting the Ultrafit Program I was a different person. I was a lean 120 pounds, but more impressive than the weight loss was the increased level of energy I was experiencing. I had a newfound outlook on life, and even though my classes were better and my abilities as a personal trainer (to lead by example) were greatly improved, I still wanted more. I knew immediately that along with finding a new body, I'd found my passion—creating and teaching a honest and effective exercise and nutrition program that I could give to my students to help them achieve and maintain what I have. And so I decided to start my own business with that goal in mind. And that was how the UltraFit Nutrition Systems was born.

In the past seven years, I have been very busy. I met and married my husband, Mike Whitmarsh, a professional beach volleyball player, and I gave birth to two incredible little girls—Jaden and Kendall. At the moment, my business has never been better. Ultrafit Nutrition Systems has expanded dramatically and now operates extensive nutrition and fitness consultation programs out of three Club One Fitness Clubs in San Diego. The success I achieved for my body ended up changing my whole life for the better.

Now when clients tell me "You can't understand what it feels like to be overweight!" I just whip out pictures of myself from seven years ago and show them how hard I've worked and how far I've come. Clients are the first to question how I stay devoted to the Ultrafit program, and the truth is that I'll never let myself go back to the way I was seven years ago. It's not just because of the way I looked. Rather, it's the way I felt about myself, and the way that others treated me. My life is now balanced and happy, and I'm driven to strive for excellence in everything I do. If I can do it, so can you. Now let's get started on the path to Ultrafitness!

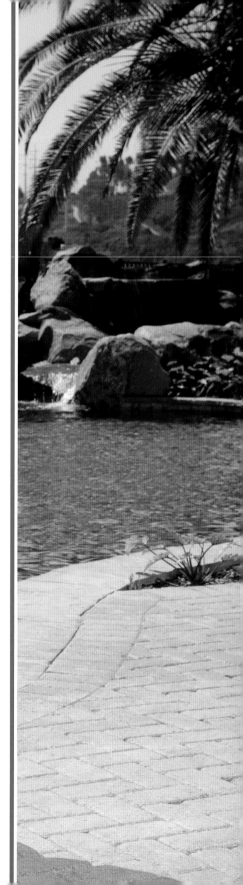

about this book

I wrote this book to give others the tools they need to become Ultrafit from the inside out. Now that means something different to everyone. My goal is to help you reach your level and idea of what being Ultrafit means to you. My passion is to share my experiences of not only my personal successs but the successes of the many clients I have helped reach their goals. This book has been designed for men and women, and I've provided three pro-grams for three different levels and stages of fitness. Let me be clear about this. This is a fitness book for individuals who cur-rently work out and are striving to become ultrafit. I get into detail in chapter 1 on what I mean about fitness levels and whether you are ready for stage 1, 2, or 3. Ideally, you should start at stage 1 and move through stage 3; each stage is a 6-week program. If you could start at stage 1 and go through stage 3 it is an 18-week program. I give detailed information so you can determine at which stage you should start. I have provided resistance-training exercises, cardio workouts, core-training workouts, and a stretch series for all stages!

In designing the programs, I tried to use as few pieces of gym equipment as possible. My goal is for people to be able to perform

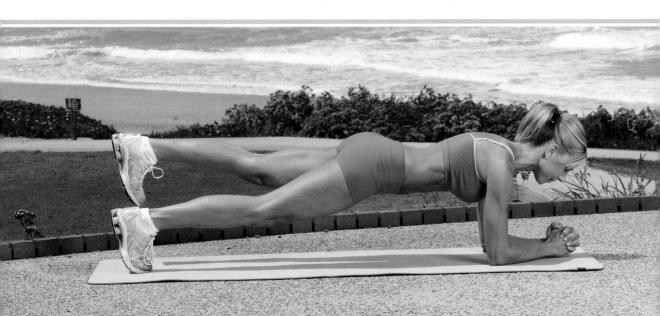

the workout routines in their home or outside with minimal equipment needed. You will need a workout bench or an aerobic step, hand weights, a jump rope, and a bike. That's it! There is a detailed calendar in each of the stages that provides a workout overview for the entire 6 weeks. I have also provided more than one hundred photos for you to see exactly what the exercises are and how to perform them correctly.

In chapter 1, I review the Ultrafit program fitness philosophy. In this chapter, I discuss my workout philosophy and the main goals and direction of this book. I follow what I call the CIC philosophy: core training, interval training, and cross training. It's important that you take the time to review chapter 2 and understand why I have you following such a specific routine. I also discuss the importance of exercise, and what kind of exercise I recommend. I also go over muscle soreness and recovery, give you the real scoop on cellulite and how to get rid of it, and explain what types of changes you can expect from your body when doing the Ultrafit program!

In chapter 2, I discuss goal setting and give you tips on how to stay motivated with your program. I ask you to sign a pledge, much like the one I made for myself at the beginning of my body transformation journey. I can't emphasize enough how important this pledge is—take it seriously! This is about challenging you and making a personal commitment to be Ultrafit!

In chapter 3, I provide the immediate steps you need to take to get on the path to becoming Ultrafit. First, I discuss resting heart rate, how to measure it, and how taking it regularly is a great way to track cardiovascular changes. Next, I discuss maximum heart rate and the training heart range you should be in for all fitness goals, including the fat-burning target heart rate range. I also show you how to assess your fitness level and determine which Ultrafit stage you should start at. The last three items in this chapter give you the specific guidelines, the tools, and the instruction you need to measure and track positive changes in your body. These changes are important to track because they will help you determine when to advance to the next level. Finally, I give you instructions on how to calculate your body fat, take measurements, and a "before" and "after" picture so you can see results and thus stay motivated!

The actual 6-week programs are outlined in chapters 4, 5, and 6. As I stated earlier, each program has a corresponding calendar that gives you a basic 6-week overview of your workout schedule everyday. You also get weekly nutrition tips to incorporate into your new program and healthy lifestyle. I designed resistance training workouts, cardio workouts, and core-training workouts for each stage. There are photographs of the specific exercises in each stage as well. The workouts in each stage are designed to progressively get more difficult, enabling you to advance through the entire Ultrafit programs (from stage 1 through stage 3). Ultimately, this book can provide you with a 6-week program, a 12-week program, or an 18-week program. But more importantly, it should help you create an ongoing lifestyle change with no definite end.

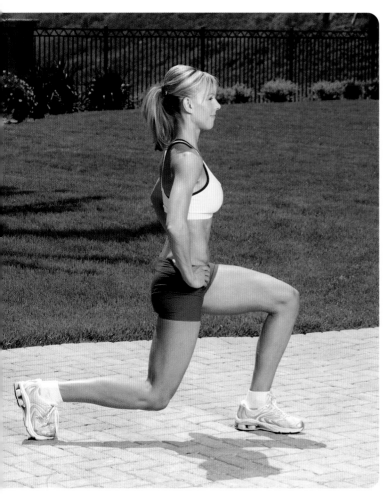

In chapter 7, I have designed a stretch series for you to follow when your workout calendar asks you to use this series. The stretch series can be applied to any stage, whether you are at stage 1 or stage 3. Remember, stretching and flexibility are just as important as any other kind of workout so don't skip this chapter!

In chapter 8, I've provided you with a comprehensive nutrition overview, much like the one I give my personal clients. I am a National Association of Sports Nutrition-licensed sports nutritionist and a certified lifestyle and weight management consultant. Even though this book is mainly dedicated to helping you reach your maximum level of fitness, I believe that proper nutrition is 70 percent of how your body looks and feels. Without the right nutrition, it doesn't matter how hard you work out; your body will never achieve the level of Ultrafitness you desire. Everyone has a different idea of what "healthy" and "fit" are, but my program has not only helped me, but also thousands of clients over the last ten years of my career. This is not a diet, but simple lifestyle changes and my tricks of the trade that work for my clients and me. Studies show that diets don't work because people abandon their diets and return to their typical lifestyle. That's why it's important to learn how to improve your lifestyle, not simply go on a diet.

Also in chapter 8, I give you my theory behind good nutrition and guidelines to follow. I will show you how to determine your nutritional and caloric needs. You will also find a sample menu and links to recipes available on the Ultrafit Web site. I am a firm believer that if the food doesn't taste good you won't want to eat it, and then your plan will fall through. You don't have to sacrifice taste to eat healthfully. I provide a sample food log to track your intake along with tons of tips, such as how to jump start your metabolism, how to eat well and exercise while traveling, and how to choose healthy meals when dining out. Last but not least, I show you how to get past those pesky weight plateaus, and how to make the Ultrafit program part of your life forever.

In chapter 9, Dr. Brian Alman gives you an amazing excerpt on mental health. Dr. Alman is not only a good friend but also a famous doctor of physiology who travels all around the world giving seminars and speaking on how to prepare yourself mentally for a healthy way of life and gain self-confidence so you can reach your own personal goals. Dr. Alman and I work with clients in conjunction with both our programs together. The results we have with our clients are instant and the percentage of our clients who keep their weight off is more than 80 percent. You have to be mentally ready to make a change or it will never happen!

So that's the gist of it! Now turn the page, get off your butt, and get started on your path to Ultrafitness!

ABOUT THE DVD

Along with this book I have put together a free 20-minute workout DVD from my fitness video, *The Ultrafit Fat-Burning Video*. The full video is a 45-minute workout, including both fat-burning cardio segments and weight training and toning intervals. I also discuss my nutrition program and include a nutrition booklet filled with menus, recipes, and all kinds of nutrition information to help you reach your fitness goals.

On those days when you only have 20 minutes free in your busy schedule to work out, put in the DVD and have a quick workout blast, including a yoga stretch and cooldown at the end. If you want the full version of *The Ultrafit Fat-Burning Video*, it can be purchased on my Web site (www.ultrafitnutrition.com).

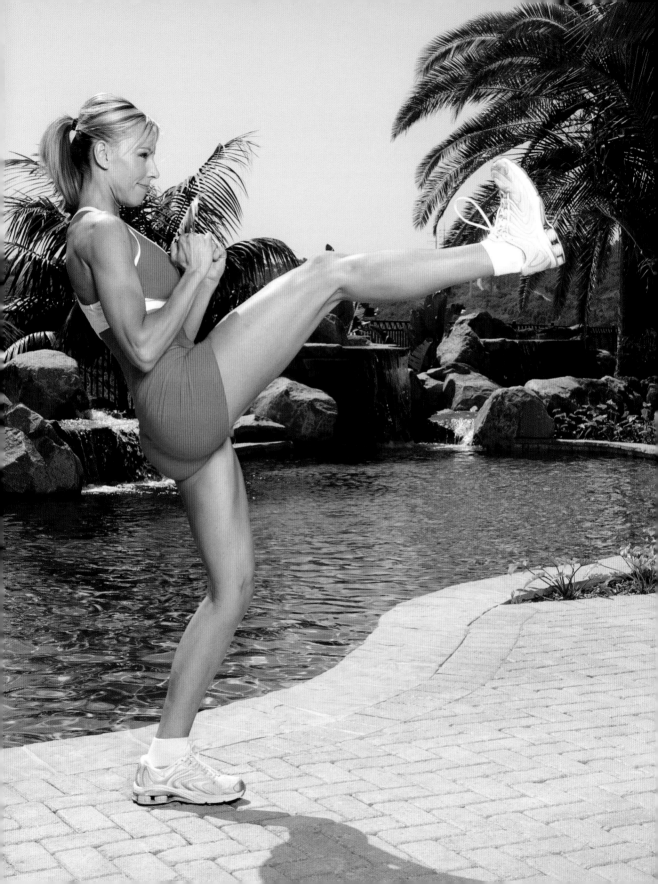

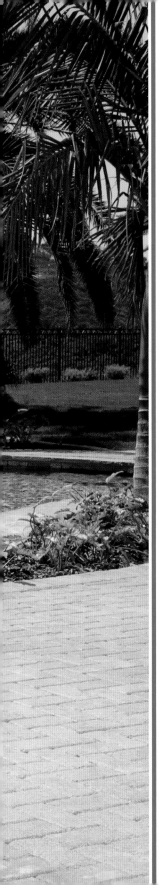

the ultrafit philosophy

There are three central concepts that form the basis of the Ultrafit program. They are:

> **Core Training,**
>
> **Interval Training, and**
>
> **Cross Training (CIC).**

I've based my own training upon these concepts, because I truly believe in their value and the importance of making changes to your body following a pattern of patient progression.

CORE TRAINING

Core training focuses on developing core strength, which is vital in any fitness regimen, because all movement originates at the core. Core training is about strengthening the muscle groups that stabilize your skeletal structure and that, in effect, link your upper body and lower body.

Core training requires that you become more aware of specific muscles, or muscle groups, especially the abdominals (including the transverse abdominus, rectus abdominus, and the internal and external obliques), the upper and lower back muscles (including the deltoids and the rhomboids). In every fitness program that I develop, I progressively introduce more difficult core movements to challenge the body. Balance challenges are a prime example of how to strengthen your core stability, even with a basic movement (e.g., standing on one leg balancing). In all my classes at Frogs Club One in Solana Beach, I throw in balance challenges. I use the BOSU (Both Sides Up) which is a half ball on a platform; it essentially throws

Greater core strength increases the stability of the pelvis and spine and improves body control and balance during workouts.

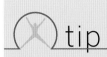

tip

If you lose weight too quickly with just dieting alone, you'll most likely lose more valuable lean muscle mass than body fat, so be sure to stick to a program that gives you no more than a two-pound-per-week loss.

you off balance, so you are forced to engage your core, exercise balls, and medicine balls. I also incorporate balance training by having my students stand on one leg while performing an exercise. This immediately forces you off balance so you have to engage your core to stay steady. This will make you stronger from the inside out!

> **REMEMBER:** You are only as strong as your weakest muscular link. My goal is to help you develop total muscular strength, wellness, and stability, without injury or fatigue.

INTERVAL TRAINING

Interval training combines brief periods of intensity (the "interval") with short periods of recovery, and then repeating the process. I constantly modify this basic template for levels of fitness ranging from virtual beginner to professional athlete.

To understand interval training, you may want to start out with an effort-to-recovery ratio such as 1:3. This might involve a hard 1-minute sprint (the "effort"), and end with a 3-minute jog or walk (the "recovery"). Depending on your ability and fitness level, you get to choose how many intervals you'd like to do in any given workout. As your fitness level improves, your ratio of effort-to-recovery should definitely change (e.g., 1:1), as well as the intensity level with which you perform the interval.

The number of repetitions and cycles you do depends on your own goals, time, and conditioning level. Interval workouts are easily adaptable to machines such as treadmills and stationary bikes. All you have to do is work out in manual mode and push the "level" button up to the desired level for the training interval and then back down for recovery. When you're outdoors, it's best to use your own "perceived exertion" scale (how hard it is on a scale of 1 to 10) to determine what you're accomplishing and how you'd like to vary your workout.

Alternating intervals of hard and easy effort increase the number of calories you burn, and improves your aerobic conditioning.

Training using interval training will provide an exciting challenge that pushes the body to change and adapt to both cardio-

Interval training is a great way to vary your training, increase your results, and get better-conditioned. It will also help you to push past a stubborn plateau, and fend off boredom by shaking up your workout and keeping things interesting.

vascular and muscular overloads. You don't have to worry about how to design your interval workouts because I have done this for you in this book. Just follow the workout calendar to guide you throughout your workouts!

CROSS TRAINING

Cross training is simply adjusting your fitness routine to include multiple activities (e.g., flexibility training, muscular strengthening, aerobic training, etc.) instead of just one. This means that your total overall fitness and performance levels improve because the same muscles, bones, ligaments, and joints aren't being stressed continuously (there's also less risk of injury as a result), and the routine stays fun and exciting.

The best results come from using different types of workouts; that's cross training!

For some of you, cross training will mean alternating between activities on a day-to-day basis (e.g., Monday: swim, Tuesday: run, Wednesday: weights, etc.), and for others it will involve multiple activities in one day's workout (e.g., 15 minutes jump rope, 15 minutes run, 15 minutes stretch, etc.). The calendar I have provided in this book will help you balance multiple fitness activities to maximize your results.

WEIGHT TRAINING

By establishing a regular exercise program with resistance (weight-bearing) exercises, you'll also build lean muscle mass.

I believe your weight training should be as intense as you are able to handle.

The same exercises that build muscle also burn fat, so the more efficient your weight training is, the less cardio you'll actually have to do. Remember in my intro how I discussed when I was forty pounds heavier? I was teaching

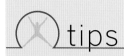

two to three high-impact aerobics classes a day back then and still not seeing the results I wanted. Weight training is thus essential to a successful weight-loss program.

MUSCLE SORENESS AND RECOVERY

This is a good time to touch on muscle soreness. A post-workout ache as well as pain in the muscles is known as delayed-onset muscle soreness (DOMS). There is a difference between being a little sore and stiff after a tough workout and being so sore that it hurts to touch your skin—so don't over-train. That said, I have included some tips to allow you to maximize your workout and avoid excessive soreness.

Lastly, it is so important to take at least one day off a week from any kind of exercise. I have clients who say, "I do take one day off! That's the day we go hiking or skiing." Excuse me, people! That is not a day off. I mean rest. No exercise at all. Your body needs rest to recuperate and rebuild. If you have a very tough week, take two days off. Over-training does you no good. In fact, it can defeat the purpose of exercising by causing excessive fatigue, hunger, water retention and weight gain, and hold you back from reaching your goals.

THE SCOOP ON CELLULITE!

Okay, so I have good news and bad news about cellulite. The bad news is that cellulite is genetically predetermined. The good news is that despite being victims of our genes, there are other factors we can control to get rid of cellulite. One factor to be aware of is dehydration. Without enough water your body is unable to properly flush toxins from your body, allowing excess toxins to collect in the fatty cells known as cellulite.

Don't be fooled into thinking that crash dieting will help either. That is the worst thing you can do for cellulite. Crash dieting puts your body into starvation mode, depositing more fat into the pockets to prepare for more meal skipping or fasting. And as if you needed one more reason not to smoke, cigarettes weaken the skin and constrict capillaries, damaging the connective tissue. That damage is often the cause of the rippling effect of cellulite!

Things that make you retain water, like sodium and diet sodas, make the appearance of cellulite look worse. So rid them from your diet and drink more water.

There is no pill, potion, or miracle cure to get rid of that nasty, cottage cheese looking junk in the trunk! The only miracle cure is good old-fashioned nutrition and exercise. It takes consistency and time but with the proper diet, and with both resistance training and cardio you can get rid of cellulite! Remember my story of the guy in the gym making fun of me because of the cellulite on my legs? Well, my cellulite is gone and I'm going to show you the exact steps I took to make my body transformation. If I can do it, so can you!

RESULTS

I'm confident in saying that if you follow this program, you're guaranteed to see positive results. When I say "results" I mean a couple of things. If you follow just the 6-week workout programs and not the nutrition program then you should see a loss in body fat, your measurements will come down, and you will become stronger and fit. If you follow the diet as well as the 6-week workouts you should see maximum physical change. The average results of my clients who are on a 6-week program are a loss of 5 to 6 percent body fat, more than 30 inches overall, and anywhere between 10 and 12 pounds. The more you put into it the more you will get out of it.

The concepts behind core training, interval training, and cross training provide the framework for the fitness program within this book, and it's vital that you understand the importance of all three. I hope that I've given you a clearer understanding of the concepts supporting my Ultrafit programs. I wish you the best of luck during this process, and I look forward to helping you achieve your health and fitness goals.

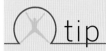

tip

Please note: *As with any exercise program, if you experience chest pains, lightheadedness or dizziness, nausea, or extreme muscular or joint pain, stop immediately and consult a physician before continuing.*

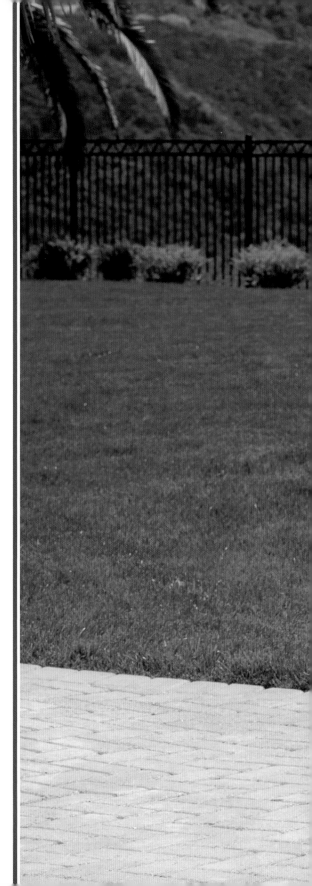

setting goals

There are four primary reasons that I see people give up on exercise programs:

Lack of results 1

Nagging injuries that won't heal 2

Boredom 3

Not setting goals 4

It doesn't have to be that way! I'm introducing you to a new way of thinking about exercise, and I'm trying to help you create a better "fit" with your lifestyle. Exercise isn't always going to be fun—but it should be challenging, provide variety, and most of all, help transform and transport your body to the level of Ultrafitness that you desire.

Ultimately, I've tried to create training programs that produce results, help prevent injuries, and keep you interested. The most popular reason my clients give for not setting goals is that they don't know how to do it well. While I can't set your goals for you, I can give you advice on how to do it yourself. I suggest you follow the "SMART" concept as outlined below:

SET SMART GOALS

This concept requires you set goals that are specific, measurable, achievable, realistic, and timely.

- **Specific goals.** I suggest being very specific and

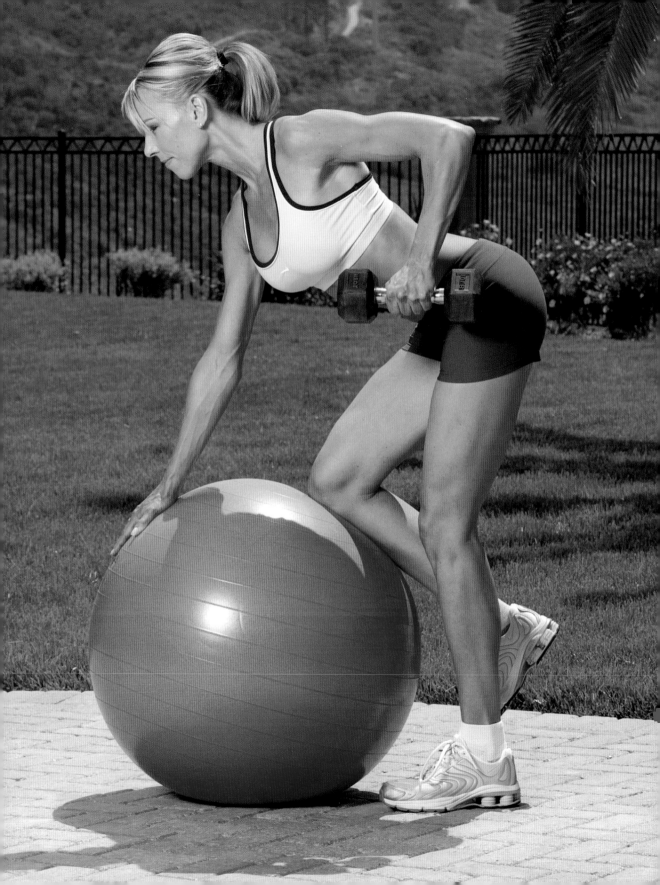

detailed when you are making your goals. For example, "After this 6-week program I want to be able to fit back into my size 6 jeans." Or, "I am going to use this 6-week program to help me train for the marathon that I am going to run in two months." Figure out what will motivate you and then set your short-term and long-term goals.

- **Measurable goals.** Nothing will keep you motivated like keeping close track of your progress and physical improvement. Make sure you begin your training by using the measuring tools I will give you in this chapter. Watching the changes in your size, BMI, and heart rate, and comparing the differences between your before and after photos that will result from adhering to the Ultrafit program will keep you going by inspiring you with the progress you are making.

- **Achievable goals.** Be true to yourself with your goals. Make sure that the goals you set are attainable—even if it might be difficult. Don't set yourself up for failure by saying you will run a marathon if you know you can't get there in the allotted amount of time you set as your goal.

- **Realistic goals.** Don't set a goal to look like someone else or a goal of unrealistic proportions. Setting realistic goals will help prevent the all-too-common tendency of starting something you can't, or don't, want to finish. For example, losing 1 to 2 pounds a week is a lot more feasible than aiming for 10 in the same period of time.

- **Timely goals.** It is important to set both short-term goals and long-term goals. A short-term goal could be losing $1^1/_2$ pounds per week and a long-term goal could be reaching your total weight loss or body fat loss targets. Make sure your goals are not too far away. Sometimes you lose track of your goals if you have too much time to reach them! I have designed this book around 6-, 12-, or 18-week schedules specifically to help make this easier for you.

But in addition to these recommendations for setting goals, I want you to consider the following points:

- **Write it all down.** Seeing your goals on paper will help keep you motivated and focused. In addition, keep a food and exercise log. The only person you're accountable to is yourself. If you're not seeing the results you want within a reasonable timeframe, review your food and exercise log and try to determine what you might need to change. If you follow a program religiously, hitting a plateau may be a sign that you need to progress to the next level, and keeping written records will help you make that decision. My clients who keep food and exercise logs are the ones who see the fastest and best results. I have a food log for you to look at in chapter 8.

- **Don't punish yourself.** Just because you slip up doesn't mean you give up. If you miss a workout or overindulge, you need to forgive and forget and get right back on track the next day. Try positive reinforcement, and start rewarding yourself when you're able to stick with the program. If you feel overly sore or exhausted, don't push it. Punishing your body when it's already sending you warning signs creates more problems than it solves. Don't get me wrong–sore muscles are going to happen (especially for you beginners), and you're going to need to learn to work through some of the stiffness and the soreness to achieve your goals. But when aches and pains grow intense, I always recommend backing off, taking a rest day—and if the pain is severe or lasts longer than three days—seeing a doctor.

- **Plan ahead.** This means creating a calendar and sticking to it. The three programs I've created for you all follow a very specific 6-week calendar. If you know you won't have time to work out after a long day on the job, get up an hour earlier and get it done in the morning. If you're not a morning person, accept that fact and stick to your plans to work out later in the day. And don't leave meal decisions to the last minute when you are tired and hungry, especially if you are trying to keep to a specific caloric intake. Grocery shop for the week ahead, and pack meals and snacks the night before so that you're always prepared for unexpected changes in your schedule.

- **Avoid over-training.** You may be tempted to stray from the 6-week programs I've developed and increase your cardio or resistance regimen under the impression that it will get you looking better even faster. You may even start skipping rest days. This will most likely only serve to decrease performance, increase fatigue, and ultimately increase the likelihood of injury. My goal is to progressively develop both your cardiovascular and muscular endurance without requiring you to spend hours working out. Getting adequate rest allows your muscles to recover and is critical to staying motivated, losing weight, and preventing injuries.

Keep exercise fresh and exciting, and always challenge the "old you." This means integrating core training, interval training, and cross training into your regimen (which I've already done for you in my 6-week programs). I want you to challenge yourself during every workout, and as you'll see upon reviewing the calendars, every week gets progressively more difficult.

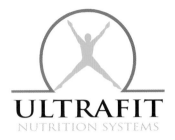

MAKING THE ULTRAFIT COMMITMENT:
SIGN THE ULTRAFIT PLEDGE

Okay, people! This is the Ultrafit Pledge. Read it thoroughly and sign your life away to me for the next 6 weeks!

Ultrafit Nutrition Program Pledge

I_____(Ultrafit participant), do hereby commit myself to following the guidelines of this challenge, and I understand that in order to achieve my goals, I must adhere to the Ultrafit program to the best of my ability. I promise to dedicate myself to at least one of the 6-week Ultrafit programs, and I take responsibility for my own actions. I understand that the program demands both time and effort, however, I will maintain a positive attitude and will not give up. I understand that if I miss a workout, it is my responsibility, and I will get back on track the next day and push myself to be the best I can be!

I will keep my food logs and dedicate myself to changing my eating habits to fit my new healthy lifestyle. I understand that this is only 6 weeks and to see maximum benefits I must be strict with my nutrition to reap the benefits of Ultrafitness!

I will dedicate myself to the 6-week program without being hard on myself or getting discouraged with my results until I take my 6-week measurements and see my "after" pictures. If I have not reached my personal goals in the first 6 weeks I will continue on for the next Ultrafit 6-week fitness stage. I will remeasure myself, take another picture, again sign the Ultrafit pledge and commit myself to another 6 weeks. I will do this until I have reached my personal goals!

I will motivate myself, and I will push myself to achieve my very best, knowing that from this effort, I have the opportunity to reap unlimited mental and physical benefits from the Ultrafit program. Through this commitment, I will work to improve myself from the inside out, as I hope to ensure a happy and healthy lifestyle that will benefit my family, my friends, and me.

Now sign and get going on your path to Ultrafitness!

Participant signature:_____ Date:_____

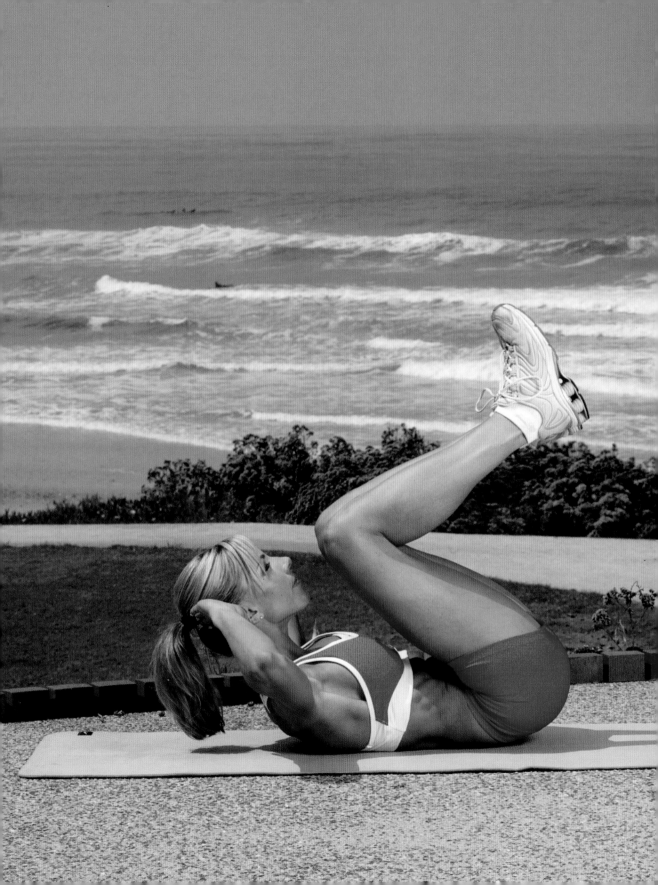

getting started

MEASURING YOUR FITNESS LEVEL
Heart Rate and Its Importance

Prior to starting anyone on a new nutrition and fitness program, I always take the time to assess his or her baseline fitness level. However, since you and I aren't interacting face-to-face, it's your responsibility to make this assessment for yourself. Your heart rate is directly related to burning fat. We will get into that in a bit. For starters, I think it's important to know about, and keep track of, three different heart rate levels:

PLEASE NOTE: Healthy men over 40 and healthy women over 50 years of age should have a medical examination and diagnostic exercise test before starting a vigorous exercise program, as should men and women of any age with health problems. If in doubt or if you have questions about your physical status, consult your physician before engaging in any vigorous physical activity or exercise test.

Resting Heart Rate

Resting heart rate (RHR) is used to help determine a person's training target heart rate, and it has proven to be an accurate method by which to track cardiovascular changes. Athletes sometimes measure their RHR as one way to find out whether they're over-training. The heart rate adapts to changes in the body's need for oxygen, such as during exercise or sleep. Your RHR represents the minimum number of heartbeats needed to sustain your body at rest, and this number raises with both age and reduced activity levels. On the flip side, this number decreases with improved aerobic conditioning. An elite athlete will have a low RHR and a person who is sedentary will have a higher RHR. The higher RHR does not necessarily indicate cardiovascular disease but more often a lack of aerobic conditioning.

Determining RHR

The RHR should be taken first thing in the morning upon waking and before getting out of bed. Attempt to do this on a day when you are not awakened by a noisy alarm that gets your adrenaline pumping. Your blood levels of adrenaline, caffeine, and other substances are lowest first thing in the morning, so this is the ideal time to take the count. It's important to note that drugs such as caffeine and those found in cold medications raise the heart rate and do not give a true indication of the resting count. Here's what you need to do:

Step 1: Use the correct fingers

Use your index and middle fingers to find your pulse. The thumb is never used as it has a pulse of its own that could interfere with a correct count.

Step 2: Locate your pulse

You can take the pulse at the neck, the wrist, or the chest. I recommend the wrist. You can feel the radial pulse on the artery of the wrist in line with the thumb. Place the tips of your index and middle fingers over the artery and press lightly.

Step 3: Count the beats

Take a full 60-second count of the heartbeats, or take it for 30 seconds and multiply by two. Start the count on a beat, which is counted as "zero."

Step 4: Record the count

The number should lie somewhere between 45 and 80.

Maximum Heart Rate and Training Heart Rate Range

Your goal during exercise is to gradually elevate your heart rate into a range (see next page) that is maintained for the 20 to 30 minutes required to assure a training effect and an adequate workout. To determine your appropriate maximum heart rate (MHR), use the following formula: MHR = 220 – age. As you increase your cardiovascular fitness, it will become more challenging to elevate your heart rate (this is a sign that your heart is working more efficiently). If your heart rate is too high, lower the level of your next aerobic routine by exercising less vigorously and minimizing your arm movements. If your heart rate is elevated by more than 10 beats per minute above your maximum, your body is working too hard and can't recover fast enough. Your recovery is when your body gains muscle and performance.

To determine your training heart rate range (THRR), use the following formula:

MHR − RHR x Target HR zone + RHR

For **moderate-intensity physical activity,** a person's target heart rate should be 50 to 70 percent of his or her MHR. For example, moderate-intensity physical activity for a 50-year-old person will require that the heart rate remains between 85 and 119 beats per minute (bpm) during physical activity.

For **vigorous-intensity physical activity,** a person's target heart rate should be 70 to 85 percent of his or her MHR. For example, vigorous-intensity activity for a 35-year-old person will require that the heart rate remains between 130 and 157 bpm during physical activity.

Fat Burning Target Heart Rate

There has been controversy over the years whether you should work out at a lower intensity or higher intensity when you are trying to burn calories and fat. Well, the truth is you will burn fat both ways, but it's the ratio of fuel sources that makes a difference. When you work out at higher intensities (60 to 85 percent MHR), although the percentage of calories coming from fat may be less than at a lower intensity, you burn more total calories overall and therefore the total number of calories from fat are higher. For example, if two people were walking on a treadmill for the same amount of time one working at 40 percent MHR and the other at 75 percent MHR the person working at the higher percentage would burn more calories from fat in the long run.

If your goals are to burn extra fat and calories, and to achieve body leanness, try to keep your heart rate mainly between 60 and 85 percent of your MHR during your cardio workouts. It's okay when you are doing a very high intensity workout to let your heart rate go higher but you should then return to your fat burning zone. Above 92 percent of your MHR, your fat oxidation rates will greatly decline.

The amount of fat you burn is also related to your fitness level. When you're more aerobically fit, your body targets more of your fat cells for energy compared to someone who is unfit. So get up and get going now!

Date	Present	6-Weeks	12-Weeks	18-Weeks
RHR (bpm)				
Moderate-intensity THRR range (50–70%)				
Vigorous-intensity THRR range (70–85%)				

Recovery Heart Rate

The recovery heart rate (RHR) is taken during the post-cooldown, for fifteen seconds, five minutes after the last aerobic activity. Multiply this number by four to determine the number of beats per minute. Recovering to 120 beats per minute in the shortest amount of time is another measurement tool for tracking cardiovascular fitness improvements. If your recovery heart rate is above 120 beats per minute for an extended period of time, then during the next activity, you should lower your workout level.

Date	Present	6-Weeks	12-Weeks	18-Weeks
Length of time to recover to 120 bpm (min:sec)				
Heart rate after full 5 min. period				

WHICH ULTRAFIT STAGE SHOULD I CHOOSE?

So now you've determined your MHR on paper, and it's time to put your fitness level to the test and determine your appropriate starting point within this program. For this, I recommend a 3-minute step test using an 8-inch step (almost any step in your home or in a gym will do). After your warm-up, step up and down in a four-count sequence as follows: right foot up, left foot up, right down, left down. (Be careful—no tripping!). Each time you move a foot up or down, it counts as one step. Count "up, up, down, down" for one set, with 20 sets to the minute. It is very important that you don't speed up the pace—keep it regular. After 2 minutes, you'll need to monitor your heart rate for the last minute. Your result should be pretty close to your age-appropriate MHR range for moderate-intensity physical activity. If your heart rate exceeds this, check with a doctor, and after she has given you the okay to return to physical activity, you should start with Ultrafit stage 1 and work your way up.

You should now have a better understanding of your individual fitness level, and you must decide where to start. Do you want to start with stage 1, stage 2, or skip all the way to stage 3? Do you need to take elements from two different programs and combine them (e.g., stage 1 weights and stage 3 cardio)? Go through the following checklist and try to make an accurate determination. And be realistic!

You should start with the stage 1 cardio program...

☐ If you have not participated in an exercise program for 6 weeks or more;

☐ If you have any medical conditions (you MUST get clearance from your physician prior to starting any exercise program) that require a beginner's program;

☐ If you are unable to maintain your heart rate within the appropriate range during the 3-minute step test; or

☐ If, after the 3-minute step test, your heart rate remains elevated above 120 bpm during recovery for an extended period of time.

You should start with the stage 1 weights program...

☐ If you have not participated in a weights program;

☐ If you have not participated in a weights program for six weeks or more; or

☐ If you have any medical conditions (you MUST get clearance from your physician prior to starting any exercise program) that require the use of light weights.

You should start with the stage 2 cardio program...

☐ If you are already participating in a cardio program equal to or more difficult than the stage 1 cardio program;

☐ If you have not participated in an exercise program for four weeks or more;

☐ If you are able to maintain your heart rate within the appropriate range during the 3-minute step test; or

☐ If you've already completed the stage 1 cardio program.

You should start with the stage 2 weights program...

☐ If you've been performing the same weights routine for 6 weeks or more with little or no change in your body composition;

☐ If you are already participating in a weights program equal to or more difficult than the stage 1 weights program; or

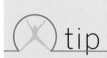
☐ If you have not participated in any weights program for four weeks or more.

You should start with the stage 3 cardio program...

☐ If you are already participating in a program equal to or more difficult than the stage 2 cardio program; or

☐ If you've already completed the stage 1 and/or stage 2 cardio program.

You should start with the stage 3 weights program...

☐ If you are already participating in a program equal to or more difficult than the stage 2 weights program; or

☐ If you've already completed the stage 1 and/or stage 2 weights programs.

DETERMINING BODY COMPOSITION

Now that you've determined your baseline fitness level and decided which program(s) to employ, you need to make an accurate assessment of your body composition. Body composition refers to the relative amounts of muscle, fat, bone, and other vital parts of the body.

Again, you're establishing a baseline from which to compare yourself to later. A scale by itself can be extremely dangerous and misleading. I have so many clients who were slaves to the scale before coming to me. It was hard to explain to them that sometimes your weight stays the same but your body fat comes down. I remember a client named Sharon, who came to see me for 6 weeks. She lost 6 percent body fat but only one pound.

To the outside world it had *looked* as though she had lost 20 pounds. Her dramatic body change was undeniable but shocking to most because of her almost insignificant weight loss. She had increased her muscle and decreased her body fat, thus the weight was not budging, but her body fat was still decreasing. It's far more important to look at changing your body from many different angles, and to provide yourself with starting points from which to determine your progress through the Ultrafit Program. This is why I had you do the heart rate tests now so you can monitor yourself as you do the workouts and see how you progress and get stronger.

Measurement Location (in)	Today's Date	6-Week Date	12-Week Date	18-Week Date
Shoulders				
Chest				
Biceps(right/left)				
Forearm (r/l)				
Waist				
Hips				
Upper thigh (r/l)				
Lower thigh (r/l)				
Calf (r/l)				

Using a Tape Measure to Calculate Body Fat

Use a non-elastic measuring tape to measure the circumference (in inches) of the body parts that appear in the chart above.Online body-fat calculators (see Ultrafit Tip on previous page) use these measurements, and your current weight, to determine your body fat. I've provided space for you to record these measurements today and again after each stage of the program.

PHOTOGRAPHIC EVIDENCE

A picture tells a thousand words, and you need to see what your body truly looks like both before and after you complete this program. Photos are the greatest way to actually visualize the progress you are making. Even if you are embarrassed wearing a bathing suit, try to wear something that allows you to see as much skin as possible. I promise you will be pleasantly surprised when your program is over. Be sure to take a front shot and a side shot.

Remember: To see maximum results in 6 weeks you need to be as strict as possible! I look back at my "before" pictures and they remind me everyday why I live the way I do. You can get there too! In fact, when you do get your pictures, I would love to see them. E-mail them to me at Cindy@Ultrafitnutrition.com if you would like. I will put them on my Web site if you'll permit me to show off your great results.

There are enough spaces for you to do all three 6-week programs. Be sure to take a front shot and side shot.

Today's Date: _____

Front View	Side View

6-Week Date: _____

Front View	Side View

12-Week Date: _____

Front View

Side View

18-Week Date: _____

Front View

Side View

stage 1 ultrafit program

Welcome to the stage 1, 6-week Ultrafit program! I am now going to explain how to use the calendar on pages 38–39 as your guide. The calendar gives a brief overview of the workouts you will be doing for the next 6 weeks. I did not get into exercise details on this calendar. All the details and pictures of the exercises will appear later in this chapter. Please note my nutritional advice and goals. For instance, each day I offer a suggested amount of water for you to drink. Again, this is only a suggestion and you can decide for yourself whether this is the right amount for you. I am trying to get you to increase your water intake each day but you should never exceed a gallon (128 ounces).

So here is how it goes: Begin with Monday as day 1. On the first day you will need to do a 10-minute warm-up of your choosing. Examples of warm-up exercises are walking or marching in place. The goal is to raise your core body temperature to prepare you for more intense exercise and to help prevent injury. Then the schedule tells you to do Weights D1 1x12 reps.

D1 stands for day 1 of the resistance training workouts I have prepared for you. 1x12 reps means you are to do 1 set of 12 repetitions of each exercise unless otherwise noted on the workout. Some exercises require you to do more repetitions. For example, the abdominal crunch—I ask you to do 1 set of 20 reps instead of the usual 12 reps for the others. Here's how to gauge the amount of weight you will need for each exercise: When you get to the last three repetitions, you should feel fatigue. If you can do more than the slated reps, then it is time to increase the weight.

I have planned two resistance training days, day 1 and day 2. Day 1 consists of chest, back, legs, and abdominals. I have also added in ski jumps to introduce plyometric (high-intensity) training and help prepare you for the intermediate and advanced workouts to come. On day 2 you will be working your shoulders, biceps, and triceps. Also in day 2, I have added cardio intervals to introduce interval training and help you burn more calories! The calendar will tell you which one to do and on which day.

You will also notice as you progress through the six weeks that I have increased your sets, reps, and the amount of cardio that I expect you to do. This is simply because you should be getting stronger and more cardiovascularly fit as the weeks go on. Now, the way to gage the amount of weight you will need for each exercise is when you get to the last three repetitions, you should feel fatigue. If you can do more than the slated reps, then it is time to increase the weight in increments of 2–5 pounds depending on your personal level of fitness level.

I have also included an extra core training workout and a stretch series. You are to do all of the workouts that are written on any given day. Also try to follow the times I have stated for each workout. You will notice that the amount of time for these cardio workouts will also increase as the weeks go by. If you can't do everything because of time or ability, don't beat yourself up. Do what you can. Studies show that 10 minutes of exercise three times a day can play a huge role in lowering triglyceride levels, lowering your risk for heart disease, and managing your weight. Just make sure that you follow the cross-training workouts that I have planned for you. It is better to cut down on the duration of a workout than not to do it at all. Remember to warm up and stretch at the end as well. Make an appointment with yourself and this book everyday for the entire 6 weeks and you won't be sorry. Now get going!

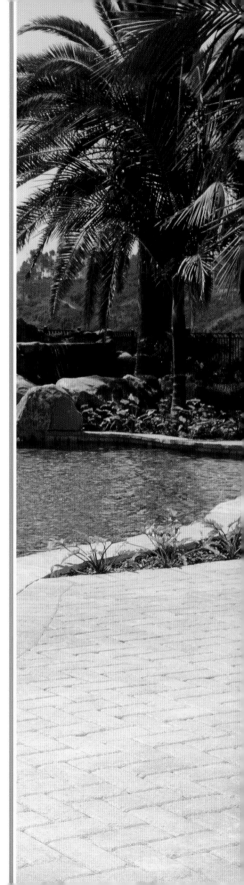

calendar

GOALS	MON	TUES	WED	THURS	FRI	SAT	SUN
WEEK 1 • Sign pledge • Take "before" pictures and measurements • Start food log • Start EFA oil and supplements (see chapter 8) • Clean out cabinets/ go grocery shopping • Write down five short-term and five long-term goals	☐ 10m Warm-Up ☐ Weights D1 ☐ 1 X 12 Reps ☐ 60 oz. H_2O	☐ 20m Treadmill Blast! ☐ Core Training ☐ 60 oz. H_2O	☐ 10m Warm-Up ☐ Stretch Series ☐ 60 oz. H_2O	☐ 10m Warm-Up ☐ Weight D2 ☐ 1 x 12 Reps ☐ 60 oz. H_2O	☐ 20m Bike Workout ☐ Core Training ☐ 60 oz. H_2O	☐ 10m Warm-Up ☐ Stretch Series ☐ 60 oz. H_2O	☐ OFF ☐ 60 oz. H2O
WEEK 2 • No candy/junk food this week • No fast food this week • Make sure you're eating 5 to 6 small meals/day	☐ 10m Warm-Up ☐ Weights D1 ☐ 1 X 15 Reps ☐ 70 oz. H_2O	☐ 20m Bike Workout ☐ Core Training ☐ 70 oz. H_2O	☐ 10m Warm-Up ☐ Stretch Series ☐ 70 oz. H_2O	☐ 10m Warm-Up ☐ Weights D2 ☐ 1 x 15 Reps ☐ 70 oz. H_2O	☐ 20m Treadmill Blast! ☐ Core Training ☐ 70 oz. H_2O	☐ 10m Warm-Up ☐ Stretch Series ☐ 70 oz. H_2O	☐ OFF ☐ 70 oz. H_2O
WEEK 3 • Write down five things you like about your body • Exercise in the morning before breakfast this week • Cut out high fat condiments and dairy	☐ 10m Warm-Up ☐ Weights D1 ☐ 2 X 12 Reps ☐ 15m Extreme Jump rope ☐ 75 oz. H_2O	☐ 20m Treadmill Blast! ☐ Core Training ☐ 75 oz. H_2O	☐ 20m Stair Challenge ☐ Stretch Series ☐ 75 oz. H_2O	☐ 10m Warm-Up ☐ Weights D2 ☐ 2 x 12 Reps ☐ 15m Extreme Jump Rope ☐ 75 oz. H_2O	☐ 25m Bike Workout ☐ Core Training ☐ 75 oz. H_2O	☐ 20m Boot Camp ☐ Stretch Series ☐ 75 oz. H_2O	☐ OFF ☐ 75 oz. H_2O

	GOALS	MON	TUES	WED	THURS	FRI	SAT	SUN
WEEK 4	▪ No alcohol for the next three weeks ▪ Go to bed 1 hour earlier three times this week ▪ Make sure you're getting 25 to 30g of fiber/day	☐ 10m Warm-Up ☐ Weights D1 ☐ 2 x 15 Reps ☐ 20m Extreme Jump Rope ☐ 80 oz. H_2O	☐ 25m Bike Workout ☐ Core Training ☐ 80 oz. H_2O	☐ 20m Boot Camp ☐ Stretch Series ☐ 80 oz. H_2O	☐ 10m Warm-Up ☐ Weights D2 ☐ 2 x 15 Reps ☐ 20m Extreme Jump Rope ☐ 80 oz. H_2O	☐ 25m Treadmill Blast! ☐ Core Training ☐ 80 oz. H_2O	☐ 20m Stair Challenge ☐ Stretch Series ☐ 80 oz. H_2O	☐ OFF ☐ 80 oz. H_2O
WEEK 5	▪ Make two new healthy recipes this week ▪ Write down five affirmations	☐ 10m Warm-Up ☐ Weights D1 ☐ 3 x 12 Reps ☐ 25m Extreme Jump Rope ☐ 85 oz. H_2O	☐ 30m Treadmill Blast! ☐ Core Training ☐ 85 oz. H_2O	☐ 30m Stair Challenge ☐ Stretch Series ☐ 85 oz. H_2O	☐ 10m Warm-Up ☐ Weights D2 ☐ 3 x 12 Reps ☐ 25m Extreme Jump Rope ☐ 85 oz. H_2O	☐ 30m Bike Workout ☐ Core Training ☐ 85 oz. H_2O	☐ 30m Boot Camp ☐ Stretch Series ☐ 85 oz. H_2O	☐ OFF ☐ 85 oz. H_2O
WEEK 6	▪ Review those short-term and long-term goals ▪ Treat yourself to some new piece of clothing ▪ Move on to the next level!	☐ 10m Warm-Up ☐ Weights D1 ☐ 3 x 15 Reps ☐ 30m Extreme Jump Rope ☐ 90 oz. H_2O	☐ 30m Bike Workout ☐ Core Training ☐ 90 oz. H_2O	☐ 30m Boot Camp ☐ Stretch Series ☐ 90 oz. H_2O	☐ 10m Warm-Up ☐ Weights D2 ☐ 3 x 15 Reps ☐ 30m Extreme Jump Rope ☐ 90 oz. H_2O	☐ 30m Treadmill Blast! ☐ Core Training ☐ 90 oz. H_2O	☐ 30m Stair Challenge ☐ Stretch Series ☐ 90 oz. H_2O	☐ OFF ☐ 90 oz. H_2O

Resistance Exercise Details

suggestions & definitions

- When selecting a set of dumbbells, the weights you choose for your stage 1 workout should allow you to complete the recommended number of reps for each exercise with moderate effort until the last three reps, when you should be feeling fatigue.

- When breathing through the exercises, exhale on the concentric (the tightening) movement and inhale on the eccentric (the release).

- When I refer to a "neutral spine" I am referring to the position of the spine. Your pelvis is not tilted, your neck is long, your abs are tight, and you look long and stable.

- When I refer to "shoulder girdle stability," I am referring to stabilizing your shoulder area by engaging or squeezing your shoulder blades and maintaining a strong upper body.

Day 1: Chest, Back, Legs, and Abdominals

EQUIPMENT NEEDED

- Hand weights or dumbbells (DB). I recommend an array of both light and heavier dumbbell weights to allow you to progress with the program and adjust the level of resistance in each exercise based on your level of fatigue. (Remember: Aim for an amount of weight that makes you fatigued in the last three sets.)
- Stability ball (55 cm is appropriate for most people. Inflate it to the point where when sitting knees are at 90-degree angle.)
- Floor space (with a mat or towel for comfort)
- Sturdy chair

EXERCISE FORMAT

- All sets and repetitions (reps) are as stated on the stage 1 calendar (unless otherwise noted).
    Example: Week I = 1 set of each exercise for 12 repetitions.
- The exercises are organized into "super-sets" of multiple exercises performed in immediate succession without any rest period in-between. Complete each series of three before moving onto the next. Example: Week 6 = sets of 15 repetitions (so you'll do each exercise in the super-set 3x15 before moving on to the next series of exercises).
- When an exercise involves switching sides, complete a set on one side and then complete the same number of repetitions on the other side.
- Don't forget to refer to the illustrations in the book for proper form and movement.

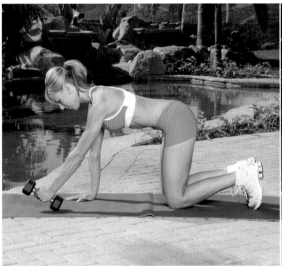 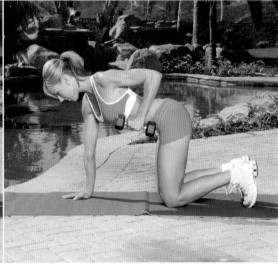

One arm dumbbell row on hands and knees (back)

1 Bring yourself to the floor and get on your hands and knees.

2 You should be in a neutral spine position, with your abs tight, and your shoulders and knees at 90 degrees.

3 Place your DB in your right hand, keeping your left arm straight and your shoulder girdle stable.

4 Initiate movement by squeezing shoulder blades together and drawing your right elbow up, bringing the DB towards your right hip.

5 Lower the DB back towards the floor and repeat.

6 Finish the reps on your right side and repeat the same number of sets on your left side. Remember to check your Stage 1 calendar for the expected number of reps for this week.

exercise 2

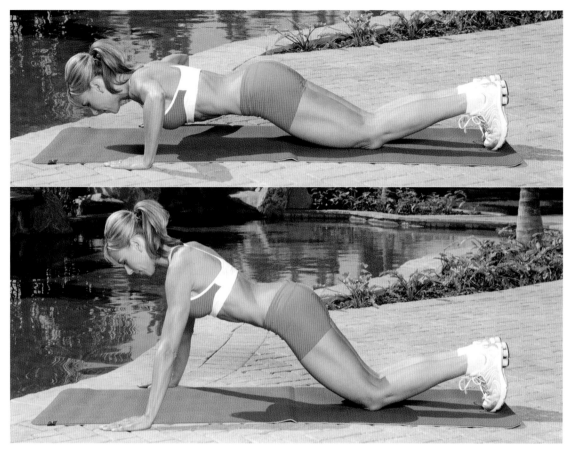

Push-ups from knees (chest)

1 Bring yourself to the floor and get on your hands and knees, your hands shoulder width apart.

2 Keep your body weight in your arms and on your hands.

3 Maintain a neutral spine and shoulder girdle stability.

4 Walk your hands away from you. The farther away you go the more challenging the exercise.

5 Once you find a position you can hold you are ready to begin the push-up.

6 Bend your elbows out to the side and lower your chest towards the floor.

7 Push yourself back up and repeat.

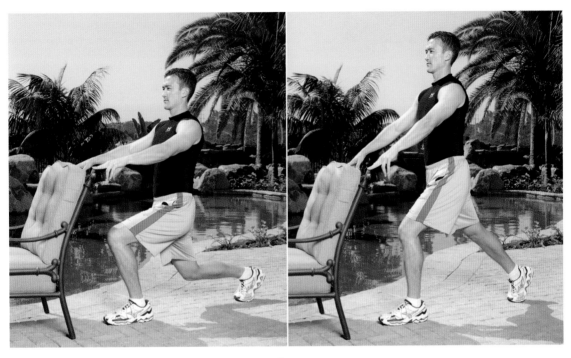

Stationary lunges holding on to a chair (legs)

1 Standing next to a chair for balance, take your left leg straight behind you so the ball of the foot is touching the floor and your heel is up and off the ground.

2 The majority of your weight should be on your front leg.

3 Bend both knees, lower your body down and push back up.

4 Keep your knees and toes going in the same direction and your upper body tall with abs tight.

5 Repeat the same number of reps on the other side.

Repeat exercises 1–3 following your stage 1 calendar guidelines of sets and repetitions

exercise 4

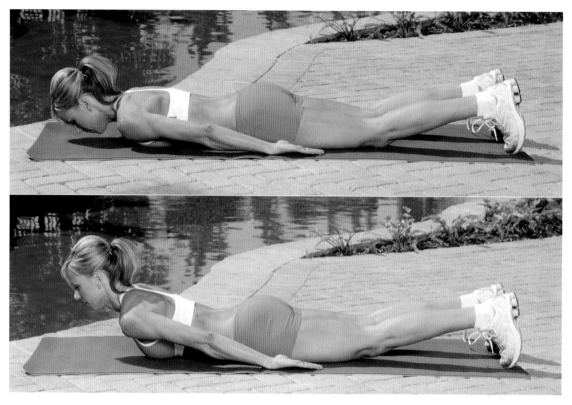

Lower back extensions (back)

1. Bring yourself down to the floor and lie on your belly.

2. Bring your hands to your sides and bring your head into a neutral spine position (looking at the floor).

3. Initiate the exercise by squeezing your shoulder blades together; lifting your head and shoulders off the floor as high as you can, keeping your feet in contact with the floor.

4. Lower yourself back down and repeat.

5. Challenge option: use a stability ball to lie on and anchor your feet against a wall.

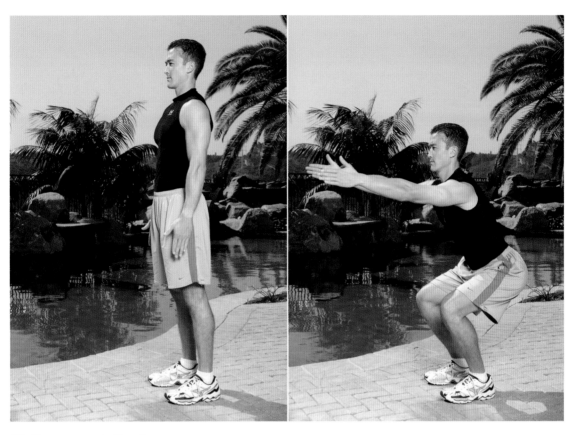

Stationary squats (legs)

1. Stand with your feet about shoulder width apart.

2. Imagine sitting on a chair, bend your knees, press your hips back, and lower yourself down.

3. Make sure your knees and toes face in the same direction and your heels stay down.

4. Keep your chest lifted and press yourself back up—repeat.

5. Do 25 total reps.

exercise 6

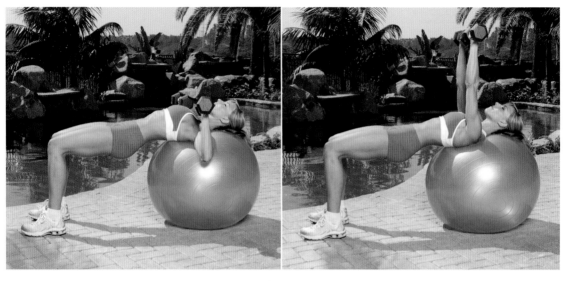

Dumbbell chest press from stability ball bridge (chest with balance)

1 Holding both DBs, sit on the ball and rest the DBs on your thighs.

2 Tuck your pelvis, lean back, and walk your feet away from the ball.

3 Keep the ball in contact with your spine at all times as you roll out.

4 The bridge is complete when your head and shoulders are supported on the ball.

5 Challenge: As you lift your hips higher in the bridge the exercise becomes more difficult.

6 Bring the DBs from your thighs and take them over your shoulders up to the ceiling.

7 Keep your hips up and don't let them sink throughout the exercise. Maintain a strong neutral spine throughout the exercise.

8 Lower the DBs by drawing your elbows out to the side.

9 Bring the DBs down towards your shoulders and press back up overhead—repeat.

Repeat exercises 4–6 following your stage 1 calendar guidelines of sets and repetitions

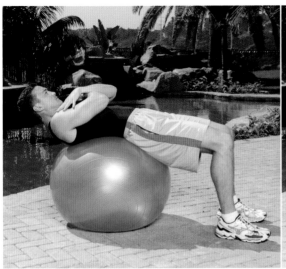 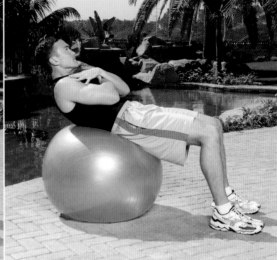

Abdominal crunches on stability ball (abs and core)

1 Sit on the ball, tuck your pelvis, lean back, and walk your feet away from the ball.

2 Walk out until your lower back is supported on the ball and the tip of your shoulder blade is touching the ball.

3 Challenge: The more "on top" of the ball you are the more difficult the exercise.

4 Either cross your hands over your chest or bring them behind your head.

5 Pull in your abs as you lift your torso up and crunch, lower yourself back down, and repeat.

6 Don't let the lower body or the ball move during the exercise.

7 Do 25 total reps.

exercise 8

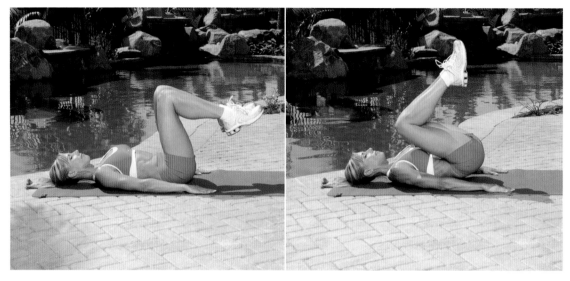

Reverse crunches on the floor (abs)

1 Bring yourself to the floor and lie on your back.

2 Bring your knees to your chest and put your hands by your sides.

3 Tighten your abs and try to lift your hips off the ground by pulling your knees towards your head.

4 Lift as high as you can, keeping your head on the floor, then control your return down. Repeat.

5 Do 25 total reps.

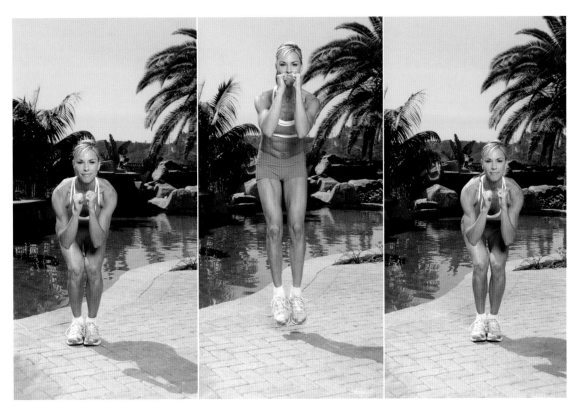

Ski jumps for 1 minute (legs and cardio)

1 Stand with your feet together, bend your knees slightly, and press your hips back.

2 Keep your feet together for the entire exercise, jump from side to side.

3 Each jump should cover 6 to 18 inches.

4 Make sure your upper body stays upright and strong.

Repeat exercises 7–9 following your stage 1 calendar guidelines of sets and repetitions

> YOU'RE NOW DONE WITH THE STAGE 1, day 1 resistance routine. Good job! Don't you feel great? Please make sure you stretch and make sure you drink plenty of water to stay hydrated! Follow your stage 1 workout calendar for your daily workout plan.

Day 2: Shoulders, Biceps, Triceps, and Core

EQUIPMENT NEEDED

- Hand weights or dumbbells (DB). I recommend an array of both light and heavier dumbbell weights to allow you to progress with the program and adjust the level of resistance in each exercise based on your level of fatigue. (Remember: Aim for an amount of weight that makes you fatigued in the last three sets.)
- Stability ball (55 cm is appropriate for most people. Inflate so when sitting knees are at 90 degrees.)
- Floor space (with mat or towel for comfort)
- Sturdy chair

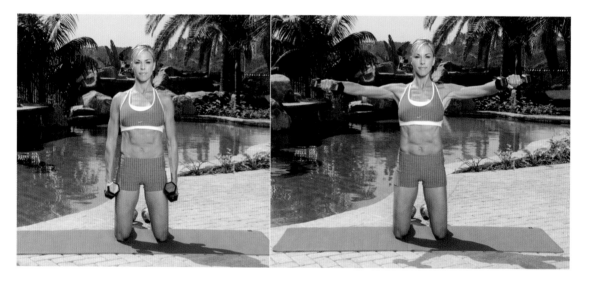

Lateral shoulder raise on knees (shoulders)

1 Bring yourself to your knees, lifting your hips up off your feet, with torso tall and erect.

2 With the DBs starting at your sides and your palms facing in, raise your arms out away from you.

3 Only bring the DBs up to shoulder height and then lower back down—repeat.

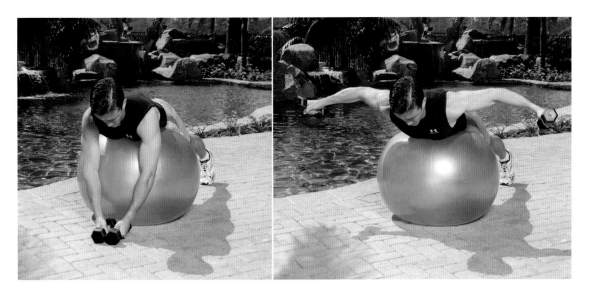

Bent over rear deltoid raise on stability ball (shoulders and core)

1 Sit on the ball with the DBs by your sides.

2 Slowly lower your chest towards your legs by hinging at the hips.

3 Keep yourself in a neutral spine position. (Don't drop your head.)

4 With your arms hanging by your sides and palms facing behind you, squeeze your shoulder blades together.

5 Draw your elbows out to your sides and up towards the ceiling.

6 Make sure your shoulders and elbows are in line with each other so you activate the rear deltoid muscle.

7 Lower the DBs back down—repeat.

exercise 3

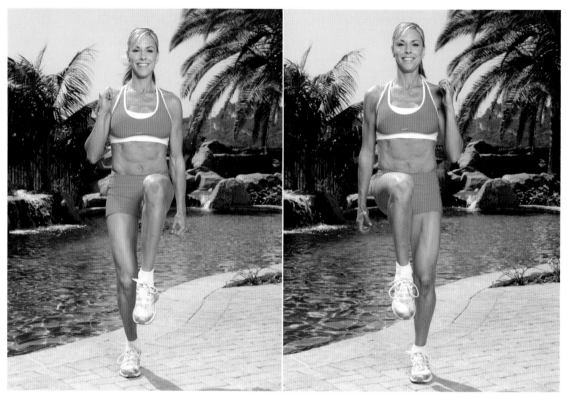

High knees for 1 minute (legs and cardio)

1 Run in place, bring your knees up as high as you can.

2 Pump those arms too!

3 This is about speed, so move and don't forget to breathe.

Repeat exercises 1–3 following your stage 1 calendar guidelines of sets and repetitions

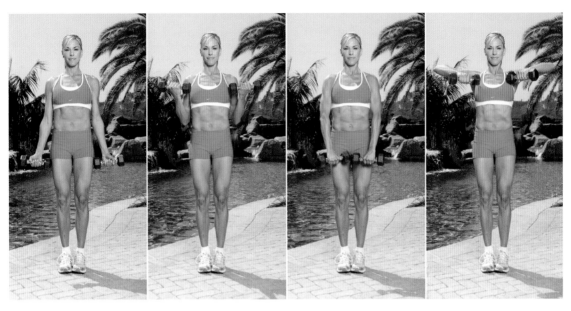

Standing biceps curl with upright row combo (biceps and shoulders)

1 Stand with the DBs in hands and your palms facing forward.

2 Begin the bicep curl by bending your elbows and drawing the DBs up towards your shoulders.

3 Lower the DBs back down and immediately flip the DBs so your palms are facing you.

4 For the upright row, draw your elbows out and the DBs up to your shoulders.

5 Lower the DBs back down and repeat from the biceps curl.

exercise 5

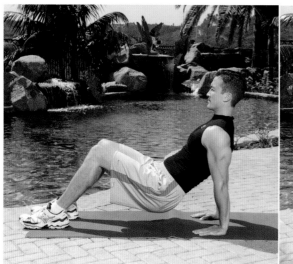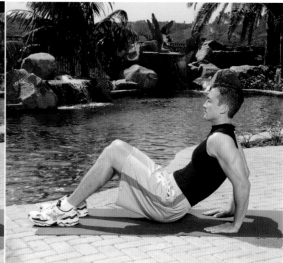

Triceps dip the floor (triceps)

1 Sitting on the floor, place your hands by your sides with your finger tips facing forward.

2 Shifting your weight onto your arms and hands, lift your hips off the floor.

3 Make sure you keep your shoulders down and back.

4 Concentrating on the back of the upper arm, bend your elbows only, and lower yourself towards the floor.

5 Straighten your elbows to lift the hips back up—repeat.

6 Challenge: Sit on the edge of a chair for a more difficult exercise.

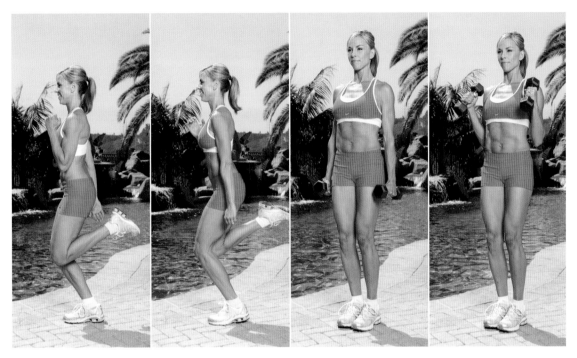

Heel kicks for 1 minute (cardio)

1 Run in place, bringing your heels to your glutes.

2 Move, move, move!

3 Pump your arms and burn some calories!

Repeat exercises 4–6 following your stage 1 calendar guidelines of sets and repetitions

Standing biceps hammer curls (biceps)

1 Stand with the DBs in your hands, palms facing in.

2 Bend your elbows bringing the DBs up towards your shoulders.

3 Return the DBs back to your sides—repeat.

exercise 8

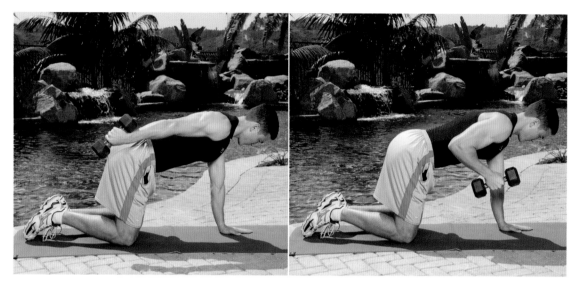

One arm triceps kickback on hands and knees (triceps)

1 Bring yourself down onto your hands and knees.

2 Your back should be flat, your abs tight, and your weight distributed over your hands and knees.

3 Place a DB in one hand, keeping the arm stabile and straight.

4 Draw the DB up so the elbow is in line with the spine and keep it there.

5 From this position straighten your elbow, tighten the triceps.

6 Bend the elbow again and "kick" the weight back up—repeat on the other side.

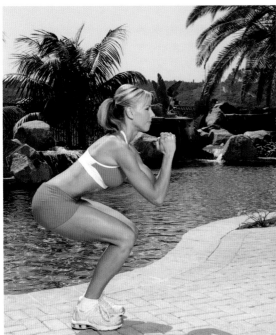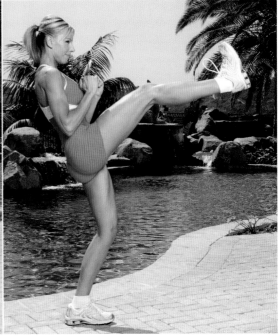

Squat with alternating forward kicks (legs/cardio) 1 minute in length

1. Stand with your feet about shoulder width apart.

2. Move into a squat by pressing your hips back and bending your knees.

3. As you lift yourself back up, kick one leg as high as you can in front of you.

4. Bring the leg back down and immediately go back into your squat.

5. Press back up and repeat the kick on the other side.

6. Keep your upper body in control and stay tall.

7. Keep your momentum going and move quickly.

Repeat exercises 7–9 following your stage 1 calendar guidelines of sets and repetitions

GREAT JOB ON YOUR DAY 2 RESISTANCE workout! How great do you feel? Please make sure you stretch and make sure you drink plenty of water to stay hydrated! Follow your stage I workout calendar for your daily work-out plan.

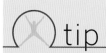

tip

Cardio Exercise Details

Stage 1: Ultrafit Treadmill Blast!

This workout can be performed outside without a machine if you don't have access to a treadmill—you just have to increase your speed if the required incline is unavailable. Try to find a hilly area so you can walk that for the second part of the workout. I like to use a treadmill because you can adjust your pace and incline instantly to keep things exciting. Using your scale of perceived exertion (scaling effort from 1 to 10), you will need to determine for yourself what slow-, medium-, and fast-paced walking means to you. When you change speeds and/or inclines, make those transitions as quickly as possible. If the workout becomes too difficult for you, bring your effort level down until you are fully recovered and then jump right back into it.

A. WARM-UP: 10 MINUTES			
TIME	FORMAT	PACE	INCLINE
2 Minutes	Walk	Slow	Flat (0%)
2 Minutes	Walk	Medium	Flat
2 Minutes	Walk	Fast	Flat
1 Minute	Walk	Slow	Flat
1 Minute	Walk	Medium	Flat
1 Minute	Walk	Fast	Flat
1 Minute	Walk	Slow	Flat

B. WORKING HARD: 10 MINUTES

TIME	FORMAT	PACE	INCLINE
1 Minute	Walk	Slow	3%
1 Minute	Walk	Medium	3%
1 Minute	Walk	Fast	3%
1 Minute	Walk	Slow	4%
1 Minute	Walk	Medium	4%
1 Minute	Walk	Fast	4%
1 Minute	Walk	Slow	5%
1 Minute	Walk	Medium	5%
1 Minute	Walk	Fast	5%
1 Minute	Walk	Medium	Flat

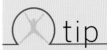

Please note: *If you experience chest pains, lightheadedness or dizziness, nausea, or extreme muscular or joint pain, stop altogether and consult a physician before continuing an exercise program.*

20-MINUTE MARK! If your workout ends here, cool down for 1 minute by walking slowly on a flat grade. You're done—now stretch!

C. WORKING HARDER: 10 MINUTES

TIME	FORMAT	PACE	INCLINE
1 Minute	Walk	Medium	3%
1 Minute	Walk	Medium	4%
1 Minute	Walk	Medium	5%
1 Minute	Walk	Medium	6%
1 Minute	Walk	Medium	7%
1 Minute	Walk	Medium	8%
2 Minutes	Walk	Fast	Flat
2 Minutes	Walk	Medium	Flat

30-MINUTE MARK! If your workout ends here, cool down for 1 minute by walking slowly on a flat grade. You're done—now STRETCH!

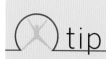

Stage 1: Ultrafit Stair Challenge

This workout requires a long set of stairs (preferably outside), that are safe to run on. I recommend visiting a local school stadium to see what's available. You can also use a step mill if one is available at your gym. I love stair workouts because the amount of calories you can burn in a short amount of time is incredible!

A. WARM-UP: 5 MINUTES

Step up and down on 1 step, right-leg leading (up-up-down-down) for 30 seconds

Step up and down on 1 step, left-leg leading (up-up-down-down) for 30 seconds

Walk up every step and walk down

Step up and down on 1 step, right-leg leading (up-up-down-down) for 30 seconds

Step up and down on 1 step, left-leg leading (up-up-down-down) for 30 seconds

Walk up every step and walk down

Step up and down on 1 step, right-leg leading (up-up-down-down) for 30 seconds

Step up and down on 1 step, left-leg leading (up-up-down-down) for 30 seconds

B. WORKING HARD: 5 MINUTES

Walk up every step and walk down

Walk up every other step and walk down

Stationary squats for 60 seconds

Walk up every step and walk down

Walk up every other step and walk down

Stationary alternating forward lunges for 60 seconds

C. WORKING HARDER: 5 MINUTES

Walk up every other step and jog down

Walk up every two steps and jog down

Push-up hold (on hands and toes) for 30 seconds

Walk up every other step and jog down

Walk up every two steps and jog down

Push-up hold (on hands and toes) for 30 seconds

Walk up every step and walk down

Step up and down on 1 step, right-leg leading (up-up-down-down) for 30 seconds

Step up and down on 1 step, left-leg leading (up-up-down-down) for 30 seconds

Repeat segments to increase workout time

ARE YOU DONE? Make sure you stretch your calves, shins, hamstrings, glutes, quads, and lower back!

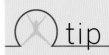

tip

Please note: *If you experience chest lightheadedness or dizziness, nausea, or extreme muscular or joint pain, I ask that you stop altogether and consult a physician before continuing an exercise program.*

Stage 1: Ultrafit Boot Camp

All you need to complete this workout is a good pair of workout shoes, and access to outside terrain (preferably on sand, grass, or a running track). The goal with this boot camp workout is to step up your cardio through interval training. Try to stick with the given exercises and time intervals to receive the maximum benefit of the workout! Good luck!

A. WARM-UP: 5 MINUTES

Walk at a relaxed pace for 60 seconds

Pick up your pace (power walk) and use your arms for 60 seconds

Walk at a relaxed pace for 60 seconds

Pick up your pace (power walk) and use your arms for 2 minutes

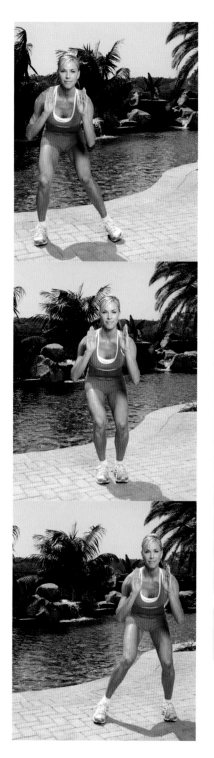

B. WORKING HARD: 5 MINUTES

Side shuffle (right leg leading) for 30 seconds

Side shuffle (left leg leading) for 30 seconds

Stop and drop! Complete as many push-ups (on your knees) as you can in 30 seconds

Turn over! Complete as many triceps dips as you can in 30 seconds

Side shuffle (right leg leading) for 30 seconds

Side shuffle (left leg leading) for 30 seconds

Stop where you are! Complete as many stationary squats as you can in 30 seconds

Keep going! Complete as many alternating forward lunges as you can in 30 seconds

Side shuffle (right leg leading) for 30 seconds

Side shuffle (left leg leading) for 30 seconds

C. WORKING HARDER: 5 MINUTES

Power walk for 60 seconds

Stop where you are! Complete as many jumping jacks as you can in 30 seconds

Stay with it! Complete as many heel kicks as you can in 30 seconds

Power walk for 60 seconds

Stop where you are! Quick feet for 30 seconds

Almost done! Complete as many high knees as you can in 30 seconds

Drop down! Hold in plank position for 60 seconds (See resistance training exercises for the photo of the plank for core)

Repeat segment to increase workout time

ARE YOU DONE? Make sure to cool down for at least a couple of minutes and stretch!

Stage 1: Ultrafit Extreme Jump Rope

This workout requires just a jump rope and you! The best part about this workout is how easily it travels with you. I always tell my clients who travel a lot to take a jump rope with them. Jumping rope is one of my favorite ways to work out. If you only have 10 or 20 minutes to do a cardio workout jumping rope is the way to go. It elevates your heart rate right away and enables you to burn a maximum amount of calories.

A. WARM-UP: 5 MINUTES

March in place for 60 seconds (no jump rope yet!)

Hop on your right leg for 30 seconds

Hop on your left leg for 30 seconds

Hop on both legs in place for 30 seconds

March in place for 60 seconds (no jump rope yet!)

Hop on your right leg for 30 seconds

Hop on your left leg for 30 seconds

Hop on both legs for 30 seconds

B. WORKING HARD: 5 MINUTES

Basic jump rope (single or double hop) for 60 seconds

No jump rope, right leg only hop for 30 seconds

No jump rope, left leg only hop for 30 seconds

Basic jump rope (single or double hop) for 2 minutes

No jump rope, jumping jacks for 30 seconds

Basic jump rope (single or double hop) for 30 seconds

C. WORKING HARDER: 5 MINUTES

Basic jump rope (single or double hop) for 60 seconds

Side-to-side jump rope for 60 seconds

Basic jump rope (single or double hop) for 60 seconds

Side-to-side jump rope for 60 seconds

Basic jump rope (single or double hop) for 60 seconds

Repeat segments to increase workout time

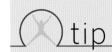

Here's a simple tip to let you know if your jump rope is the appropriate length for you: When standing on the middle of the rope, the ends should reach up directly under your armpits.

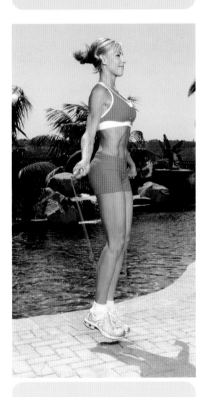

ARE YOU DONE? Make sure to cool down and stretch!

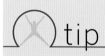

Stage 1: Ultrafit Bike Workout

You will need a stationary bike, a Spin Cycle, or an outside bike to complete this workout. If you're using an outside bike you can adjust the tension on your bike to reflect the workout intervals. For example, when the workout asks you to climb at a medium pace, crank up the tension until it makes you stand up and cycle. That way you are approximating a climb. You'll need to use your scale of perceived exertion (scaling effort from 1 to 10) combined with adjusting the bike tension on a scale of 1 to 10 throughout the workout. If the workout becomes too difficult for you, bring your effort level down until you are fully recovered and then jump right back into it. Remember to check your heart rate regularly and maintain the appropriate heart rate zone (I always recommend using a heart rate monitor).

A. WARM-UP: 10 MINUTES			
TIME	FORMAT	PACE	TENSION
1 Minute	Seated Cycle	Slow	None
1 Minute	Seated Cycle	Medium	None
1 Minute	Seated Cycle	Fast	None
1 Minute	Seated Cycle	Slow	None
1 Minute	Seated Cycle	Medium	None
1 Minute	Seated Cycle	Fast	None
1 Minute	Seated Cycle	Slow	None
1 Minute	Seated Cycle	Medium	None
1 Minute	Seated Cycle	Fast	None
1 Minute	Seated Cycle	Slow	None

B. WORKING HARD: 10 MINUTES

TIME	FORMAT	PACE	TENSION
1 Minute	Seated Cycle	Slow	2%
1 Minute	Seated Cycle	Medium	2%
1 Minute	Seated Cycle	Fast	2%
1 Minute	Seated Cycle	Slow	4%
1 Minute	Seated Cycle	Medium	4%
1 Minute	Seated Cycle	Fast	4%
1 Minute	Seated Cycle	Slow	6%
1 Minute	Seated Cycle	Medium	6%
1 Minute	Seated Cycle	Fast	6%
1 Minute	Seated Cycle	Medium	None

20-MINUTE MARK! If your workout ends here, cool down for 1 minute by pedaling slowly with no tension. You're done—now stretch!

C. WORKING HARDER: 10 MINUTES

TIME	FORMAT	PACE	TENSION
1 Minute	Seated Cycle	Slow	6%
1 Minute	Seated Cycle	Medium	6%
1 Minute	Seated Cycle	Fast	6%
1 Minute	Climbing Cycle	Medium	8%
1 Minute	Climbing Cycle	Medium	8%
1 Minute	Climbing Cycle	Medium	8%
1 Minute	Seated Cycle	Slow	6%
1 Minute	Seated Cycle	Medium	6%
1 Minute	Seated Cycle	Fast	6%
1 Minute	Climbing Cycle	Medium	10%

30-MINUTE MARK! If your workout ends here, cool down for 1 minute by pedaling slowly with no tension. You're done—now stretch!

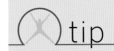

tip

Please note: If you experience chest pains, lightheadedness or dizziness, nausea, or extreme muscular or joint pain, I ask that you stop altogether and consult a physician before continuing an exercise program.

Ultrafit Core Training Details

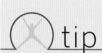

tip

It's extremely important that you both breathe correctly and, at the same time, properly draw in your abdominal muscles prior to engaging in any of these exercises.

You have a "corset" that wraps around your abdomen and back called the transverse abdominus, and once you learn to isolate the transverse abdominus, you'll be on your way to a stronger back and a flatter tummy. Imagine a string attached to the inside of your belly button. Take a deep breath through your nose and exhale through your mouth, while at the same time pulling the string towards your spine and drawing your belly button in. You should still be able to breathe correctly while holding this muscle in position.

EQUIPMENT NEEDED

- Stability ball

EXERCISE FORMAT

- There are different super-sets of exercises (exercises to be performed back to back), each to be completed three times before moving onto the next super-set.

suggestions and definitions

This abdominal workout has been designed to target your entire "core" area. When I mention an "isometric" move (e.g., "V-sit isometric hold"), it actually refers to no movement at all. Isometric training requires you to sustain a muscle contraction over a given period of time, and there are no repetitions required. The end result of isometric training is that the muscle begins to recruit and activate more motor units to help maintain this contraction, which are then forced to contract continuously, time after time, thus maturing the entire muscle very quickly.

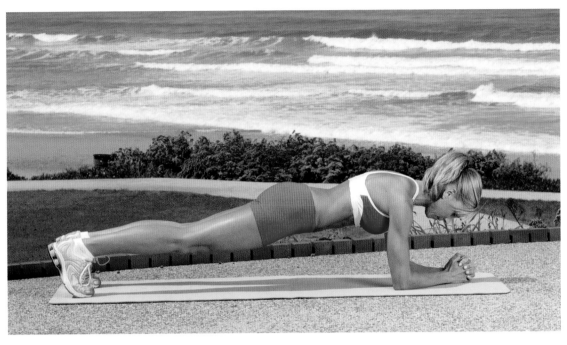

Plank hold from forearms and toes for 30 seconds in length

1 Get down on the floor on your hands and knees.

2 Bring yourself down so that you are resting on your forearms.

3 Make sure your shoulders are directly over your elbows and clasp your hands together.

4 Tighten up those abs and keep your spine long.

5 Extend both your legs so that your knees are off the ground and your toes are supporting you.

6 Your body should be straight from the tip of your head all the way through to your feet.

7 Make sure you don't drop into your shoulders or arch your back; maintain shoulder girdle stability.

8 The 30-second hold doesn't begin until you're up in the plank.

exercise 2

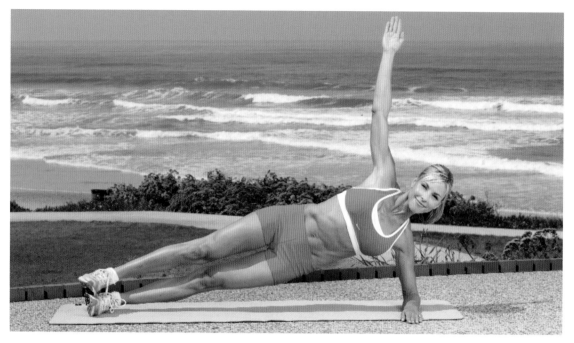

Side plank 30 seconds in length

1. Bring yourself into the forearm plank hold as described earlier.

2. Bring your forearms together so they are touching, parallel to each other, and each hand is touching the opposite elbow.

3. Roll yourself onto your right elbow with your shoulder directly over the elbow.

4. You'll now be looking at the wall instead of the floor.

5. Make sure your hips are stacked on top of each other and your feet are stacked on top of each other.

6. Extend your left arm up to the ceiling, opening your chest.

7. Contract your abdominals and breathe.

8. The 30-second hold doesn't begin until you're up in the plank on your right elbow.

9. Repeat on the left side for 30 seconds.

Repeat exercises 1 and 2 for 3 sets

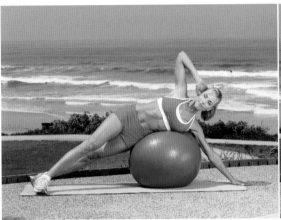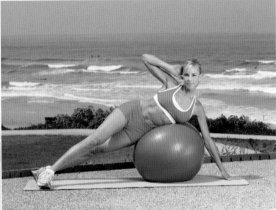

Side crunches on stability ball; 25 reps

1 Get on your knees with the stability ball touching your hips directly in front of you.

2 Roll yourself forward over the stability ball, engaging your lower back and keeping your chest lifted.

3 Your feet should be about 12 inches apart.

4 Your hips should be pushing into the stability ball and your head and shoulders should be higher than the stability ball.

5 Slowly roll yourself onto your right hip, making sure you keep the hips stacked and the spine long.

6 Your feet will then be staggered with your left foot slightly in front of the right foot.

7 Bring your left hand behind your head and your right hand can help with balance if needed, or bring the right hand behind your head as well.

8 From here, bring your left shoulder towards your hips, lower back down and repeat for 25 reps.

9 The stability ball should not move during the exercise.

10 Repeat on the left hip.

exercise 4

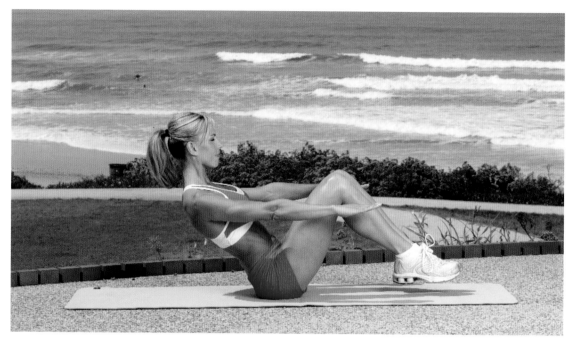

V-sit isometric hold on floor for 30 seconds in length

1 Sit on the floor bringing your knees into your chest with your feet off the floor.

2 Make sure your chest is lifted, your shoulders are back, and those abs are really tight.

3 Keep your back as straight as possible.

4 Reach your arms straight in front of you and hold.

5 Your 30 seconds doesn't start until you are balanced in the "V" position.

6 **N O T E :** If this hurts your back in any way, keep your feet on the ground and hold that position until you are strong enough to lift your feet.

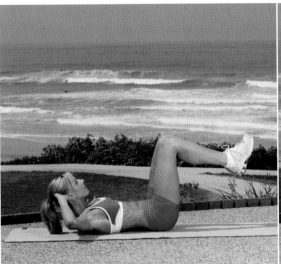 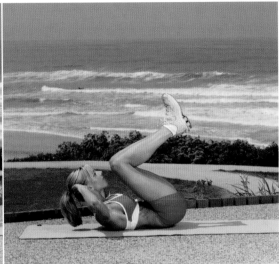

Combo abdominal crunches: 15 reps

1 Lie on the floor with your knees up towards your chest and your hands cradling your head.

2 Keep your knees at a 90-degree angle and make sure your elbows are open wide.

3 Pulling that belly button in really tight, bring your chest up without pulling on your neck, and at the same time bring your knees in towards your chest.

4 Lower yourself back to the floor, without resting, and repeat for 15 reps.

Repeat exercises 3 through 5, for 3 sets

GREAT JOB! NOW REMEMBER TO STRETCH!
Lying on the ball with your arms stretched out to your sides and your feet planted on the floor is a great way to stretch out your abdominal area!

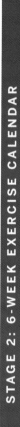

CHAPTER 5

stage 2 ultrafit program

Welcome to the stage 2, 6-week Ultrafit program. If you have already finished the stage 1 program, then congratulations! If you have skipped the stage 1 program and are beginning with the stage 2 program, then let's get started!

The calendar on pages 74–75 gives a brief overview of the workouts you will be doing for the next 6 weeks. Just as in the stage 1 program, I did not get into exercise details on this calendar. All the details and pictures of the exercises, as well as my nutritional advice and goals for you, follow in this chapter.

If you have done the stage 1 program, I would like you to begin again like you did 6 weeks ago and re-sign the pledge and follow the stage 2 nutritional advice as before. For each day, I give a suggested amount of water for you to drink. Again, this is only a suggestion and you can decide for yourself whether this is the right amount for you. I am trying to get you to increase your water intake each day but you should never exceed a gallon (128 ounces). So here is how it goes: begin with Monday as day 1. You will need to do Weights D1 2x12 reps.

> D1 stands for Day 1 of the resistance training workouts I have prepared for you. 2x12 reps means you are to do 2 sets of 12 repetitions of each exercise unless otherwise noted on the workout. Some exercises require you to do more repetitions. The calendar also tells you to do the 20 minute treadmill workout after your weight workout.

I have planned two resistance-training days, day 1 and day 2. Day 1 consists of chest, back, legs, and abdominals. I have also added in walking lunges with plyometric jumps to step up your plyometric (high-intensity) training and help prepare you for the advanced workouts to come. On day 2 you will be working your shoulders, biceps, triceps, and core as well as doing cardio intervals to introduce interval training and help you burn more calories! The calendar will tell you which one to do and on which day.

As you progress through the 6 weeks you will increase your sets, reps, and the amount of cardio that I expect you to do. This is simply because you should be getting stronger and more fit as the weeks go on.

I have also included an extra core training workout and a stretch series. You are to do all of the workouts that are written for any given day. Also try to follow the times I have stated for each workout. You will notice that the amount of time for these cardio workouts will also increase as the weeks go by. If you can't do everything, don't beat yourself up! Do what you can. Studies show that 10 minutes three times a day can play a huge roll in lowering triglyceride levels, lowering your risk for heart disease, and with weight management. You have to devote time to reach your goals! Now get going and have fun!

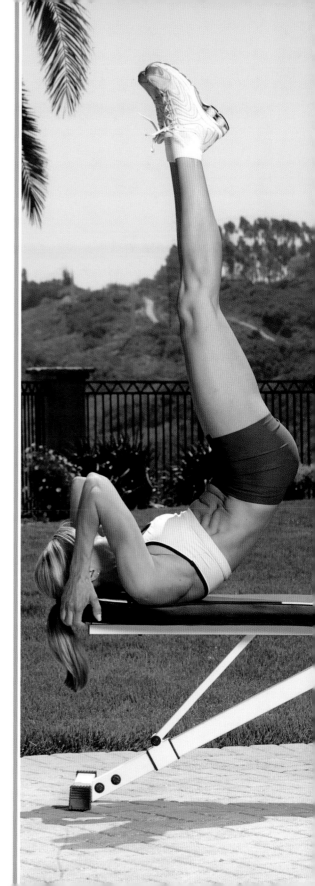

calendar

	GOALS	MON	TUES	WED	THURS	FRI	SAT	SUN
WEEK 1	■ Sign pledge ■ Schedule check-up (if you have not already done so in Stage 1) ■ Take "before" pics and measurements ■ Start food log ■ Start FEA oil and supplements (see chapter 8) ■ Clean out cabinets/go grocery shopping ■ Write down five short-term and five long-term goals	□ Weights D1 □ 2 x 12 Reps □ 20m Treadmill Blast! □ 90 oz. H_2O	□ Weights D2 □ 2 x 12 Reps □ 20m Stair Challenge □ 90 oz. H_2O	□ 20m Extreme Jump Rope □ Core Training □ Stretch Series □ 90 oz. H_2O	□ Weights D1 □ 2 x 12 Reps □ 20m Boot Camp □ 90 oz. H_2O	□ Weights D2 □ 2 x 12 Reps □ 20m Bike Workout □ 90 oz. H_2O	□ 20m Sprint Intervals □ Core Training □ Stretch Series □ 90 oz. H_2O	□ OFF □ 90 oz. H_2O
WEEK 2	■ No candy/junk food this week ■ No fast food this week ■ Make sure you're eating 5 or 6 small meals/day	□ Weights D1 □ 2 x 15 Reps □ 25m Boot Camp □ 100 oz. H_2O	□ Weights D2 □ 2 x 15 Reps □ 25m Bike Workout □ 100 oz. H_2O	□ 25m Sprint Intervals □ Core Training □ Stretch Series □ 100 oz. H_2O	□ Weights D1 □ 2 x 15 Reps □ 25m Treadmill Blast! □ 100 oz. H_2O	□ Weights D2 □ 2 x 15 Reps □ 25m Stair Challenge □ 100 oz. H_2O	□ 25m Extreme Jump Rope □ Core Training □ Stretch Series □ 100 oz. H_2O	□ OFF □ 100 oz. H_2O
WEEK 3	■ Write down five things you like about your body ■ Exercise in the morning before breakfast this week ■ Cut out high-fat condiments and dairy	□ Weights D1 □ 3 x 15 Reps □ 30m Treadmill Blast! □ 110 oz. H_2O	□ Weights D2 □ 3 x 15 Reps □ 30m Stair Challenge □ 110 oz. H_2O	□ 30m Extreme Jump Rope □ Core Training □ Stretch Series 110 oz. H_2O	□ Weights D1 □ 3 x 15 Reps □ 30m Boot Camp □ 110 oz. H_2O	□ Weights D2 □ 3 x 15 Reps □ 30m Bike Workout □ 110 oz. H_2O	□ 30m Sprint Intervals □ Core Training □ Stretch Series □ 110 oz. H_2O	□ OFF □ 110 oz. H_2O

	GOALS	MON	TUES	WED	THURS	FRI	SAT	SUN
WEEK 4	■ No alcohol for the next three weeks ■ Go to bed 1 hour earlier three times this week ■ Make sure you're getting 25 to 30g of fiber/day	☐ Weights D1 ☐ 3 x 20 Reps ☐ 30m Boot Camp ☐ 120 oz. H_2O	☐ Weights D2 ☐ 3 x 20 Reps ☐ 30m Bike Workout ☐ 120 oz. H_2O	☐ 30m Sprint Intervals ☐ Core Training ☐ Stretch Series ☐ 120 oz. H_2O	☐ Weights D1 ☐ 3 x 20 Reps ☐ 30m Treadmill Blast! ☐ 120 oz. H_2O	☐ Weights D2 ☐ 3 x 20 Reps ☐ 30m Stair Challenge ☐ 120 oz. H_2O	☐ 30m Extreme Jump Rope ☐ Core Training ☐ Stretch Series ☐ 120 oz. H_2O	☐ OFF ☐ 120 oz. H_2O
WEEK 5	■ Make two new healthy recipes this week ■ Write down five affirmations	☐ Weights D1 ☐ 3 x 15, 12, 10 ☐ 30m Treadmill Blast! ☐ 120 oz. H_2O	☐ Weights D2 ☐ 3 x 15, 12, 10 ☐ 30m Stair Challenge ☐ 120 oz. H_2O	☐ 30m Extreme Jump Rope ☐ Core Training ☐ Stretch Series ☐ 120 oz. H_2O	☐ Weights D1 ☐ 3 x 15, 12, 10 ☐ 30m Boot Camp ☐ 120 oz. H_2O	☐ Weights D2 ☐ 3 x 15, 12, 10 ☐ 30m Bike Workout ☐ 120 oz. H_2O	☐ 30m Sprint Intervals ☐ Core Training ☐ Stretch Series ☐ 120 oz. H_2O	☐ OFF ☐ 120 oz. H_2O
WEEK 6	■ Review your short-term and long-term goals ■ Treat yourself to some new piece of clothing ■ Move on to the next level!	☐ Weights D1 ☐ 3 x 12, 10, 8 ☐ 30m Boot Camp ☐ 120 oz. H_2O	☐ Weights D2 ☐ 3 x 12, 10, 8 ☐ 30m Bike Workout ☐ 120 oz. H_2O	☐ 30m Sprint Intervals ☐ Core Training ☐ Stretch Series ☐ 120 oz. H_2O	☐ Weights D1 ☐ 3 x 12, 10, 8 ☐ 30m Treadmill Blast! ☐ 120 oz. H_2O	☐ Weights D2 ☐ 3 x 12, 10, 8 ☐ 20m Stair Challenge ☐ 120 oz. H_2O	☐ 30m Extreme Jump Rope ☐ Core Training ☐ Stretch Series ☐ 120 oz. H_2O	☐ OFF ☐ 120 oz. H_2O

Resistance Exercise Details

suggestions & definitions

- When selecting a set of dumb-bells for your stage 2 workout, it should be somewhat hard to complete the recommended number of reps for each exercise. Also the last three reps should be extremely difficult to finish. You want to fatigue the muscle!

- When breathing through the exercises, exhale on the concentric (the contraction) movement and inhale on the eccentric (the release).

- When I refer to a "neutral spine" I am referring to the position of the spine. The pelvis is not tilted, the neck is long, the abs are tight, and you look long and stable.

- When I refer to "shoulder girdle stability" I am referring to stabilizing your shoulder area by engaging or squeezing your shoulder blades and maintaining a strong upper body.

Day 1: Chest, Back, Legs, and Abdominals

EQUIPMENT NEEDED

- Hand weights or dumbbells (DB). I recommend an array of both light and heavier dumbbell weights to allow you to progress with the program and adjust the level of resistance in each exercise based on your level of fatigue. (Remember: Aim for an amount of weight that makes you fatigued in the last three sets.)

- Stability ball (55 cm is appropriate for most people). (Inflate the ball to the point that when sitting your knees are bent at 90 degree angles.)

- Floor space (with a mat or towel for comfort)

- Exercise bench or aerobic step

EXERCISE FORMAT

- All sets and repetitions (reps) are as stated on the stage 2 calendar (unless otherwise noted).
  Example: Week 1 = 2 sets of each exercise for 12 repetitions.

- The exercises are organized into "super-sets," i.e., a group of exercises done in quick succession without a break period in-between. Complete each series of three before moving on to the next. Example: Week 6 = 3 sets of 15, 12, 10 repetitions (so you'll do each super-set three times before moving on to the next.)

- When the set repetitions are stated as a pyramid (e.g., 15, 12, 10) your corresponding weight should go up as the reps go down (e.g., 10 lbs, 12 lbs, 15 lbs).

- When an exercise involves switching sides, complete a set on one side and then complete the same number of repetitions on the other side.

- Don't forget to refer to the illustrations in the book for proper form and movement.

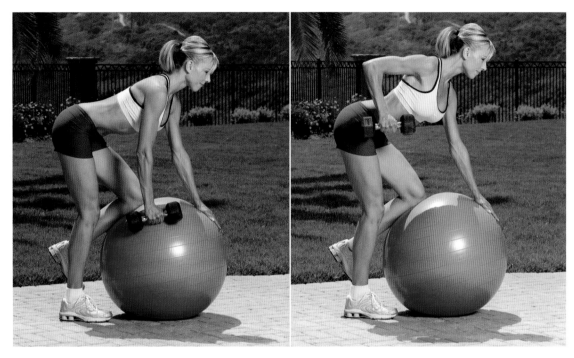

One arm dumbbell row on stability ball (back and core)

1 Take a DB in your left hand. Keep your left foot on the floor and put your right hand and right knee on top of the ball.

2 Bend over and keep your spine in a neutral position; let your left arm and the DB reaching towards the floor.

3 Initiate the row by squeezing your shoulder blades together and draw your left elbow up and back towards your hip.

4 Lower the DB back towards the floor. Finish the reps and repeat on the other side.

exercise 2

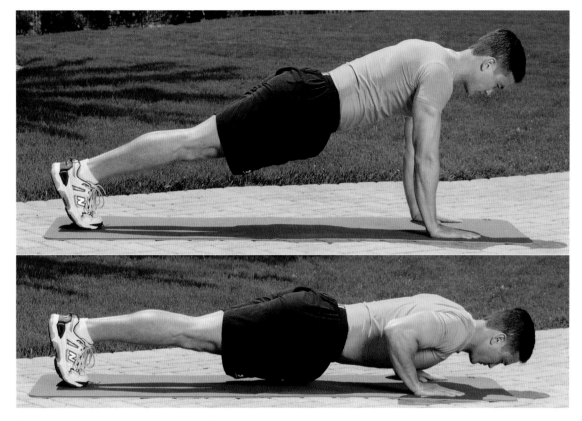

Push-ups from knees or toes (chest)

1. Bring yourself to the floor and get on your hands and knees, with your hands shoulder width apart.

2. Support your body weight in your arms and on your hands.

3. Maintain neutral spine and shoulder girdle stability.

4. Walk your hands away from you while lifting your knees off the floor so your body is parallel to the ground.

5. Once you find a position you can hold, you are ready to begin the push-up.

6. Bend your elbows out to the side and lower your chest towards the floor.

7. Push yourself back up and repeat.

8. **NOTE:** If you find it difficult to do the push-up from your toes, you can always drop down to your knees to finish the reps.

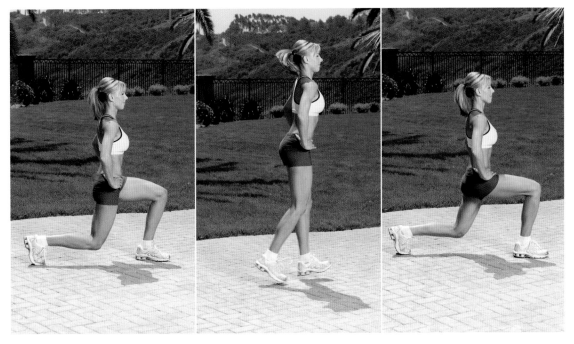

Plyometric lunge jump (legs and cardio)

1 Start with a split stance position. Stand on your left leg and extend your right leg behind you with your back heel up.

2 Your upper body should be in control with your hands on your hips.

3 Bend both knees and press your hips back slightly.

4 Jump and switch leg positions with the right leg in front and the left leg in back.

5 Bend your knees again and repeat.

6 Do 30 reps total—15 on each side.

Repeat exercises 1–3 following your stage 2 calendar guidelines of sets and repetitions

exercise 4

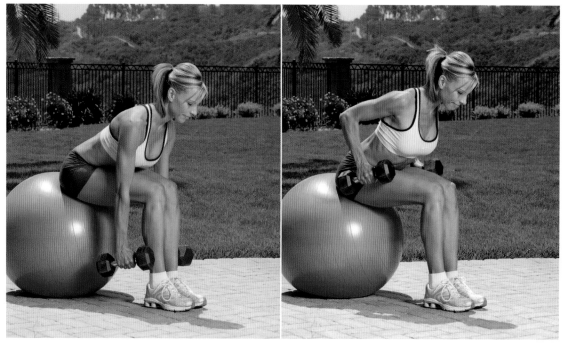

Seated bent-over dumbbell row on stability ball (back and core)

1   Sit on the ball with the DBs by your sides.

2   Slowly lower your chest towards your legs by hinging at the hips.

3   Keep yourself in a neutral spine position. (Don't drop your head.)

4   With your arms hanging by your sides and your palms facing behind you, squeeze your shoulder blades together.

5   Draw your elbows out to your sides and up towards the ceiling.

6   Lower the DBs back down—repeat.

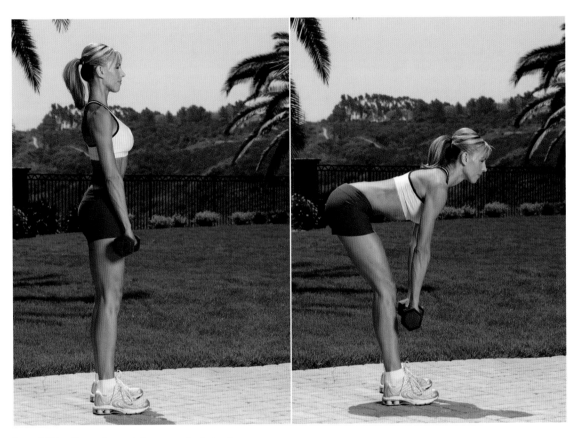

Dead lifts (legs, hamstrings, and glutes)

1 Start by standing with your feet shoulder width apart, DBs in your hands, palms facing your legs.

2 With your knees soft, keep your spine perfectly straight and hinge (or bend over) at the hips.

3 Lower the DBs down toward the floor.

4 Only go as low as you can while keeping your spine straight.

5 Engage the hamstrings, tighten your glutes, and lift your torso back to an upright position; repeat.

exercise 6

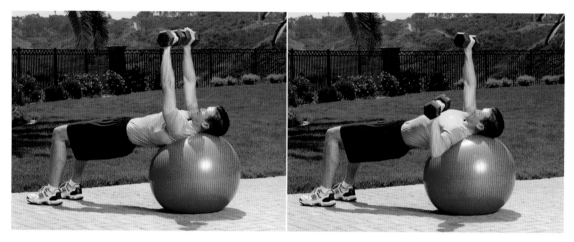

Stability ball bridge with alternating dumbbell chest press (chest and core)

1 Holding both DBs, sit on the ball and rest the DBs on your thighs.

2 Tuck your pelvis, lean back, and walk your feet away from the ball.

3 Keep the ball in contact with your spine at all times as you roll out.

4 The bridge is complete when your head and shoulders are supported on the ball.

5 Challenge: As your lift your hips higher in the bridge, the exercise gets more difficult.

6 Bring the DBs from your thighs and take them over your shoulders up to the ceiling.

7 Keep your hips up and stationary. Maintain a strong neutral spine throughout the exercise.

8 Lower the left DB toward your shoulder by drawing your elbow out to the side and down.

9 The right arm stays up over the shoulder.

10 Press the left DB back up to the ceiling, stabilize, and repeat with the right arm.

11 Alternate left and right arms until the reps are complete.

Repeat exercises 4–6, following your stage 2 calendar guidelines of sets and repetitions

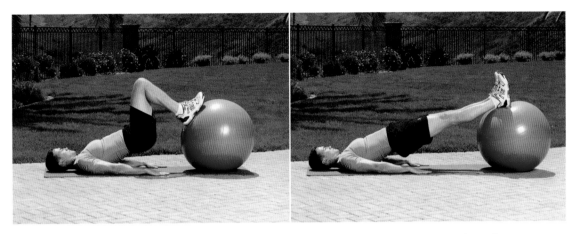

Glute and hamstring curls with stability ball; 30 reps (legs, hamstrings, glutes, and core)

1 Lie on the floor with your heels on top of the ball and your hands by your sides.

2 Gently push your heels into the ball, lifting your hips up off the floor and squeezing your glutes.

3 Keeping your hips up, bend your knees and draw your heels into your glutes.

4 Push your heels back out and straighten your legs.

5 Lower your hips but don't let them touch the ground.

6 Lift your hips back up and repeat the hamstring curl.

7 Maintain a strong neutral spine throughout the entire exercise.

8 Do a total of 30 reps.

exercise 8

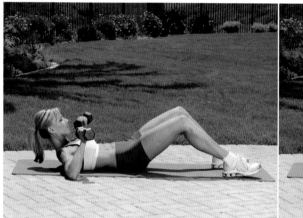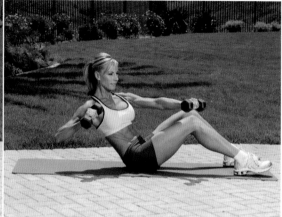

Alternating abdominal cross punches; 30 reps (abdominals)

1 Lie on the floor with your knees bent and your feet flat on the floor.

2 Pull your belly button into your spine and keep it pulled in throughout the entire exercise.

3 Exhale and lift your head and shoulders off the floor; hold.

4 You begin here with your hands in front of you.

5 Punch your right arm toward your left knee, lifting your torso up off the floor and toward the left knee.

6 Lower your torso to the floor and repeat the punch with the left arm to the right knee.

7 Keep your neck in a neutral position.

8 Do a total of 30 total reps, 15 on each side.

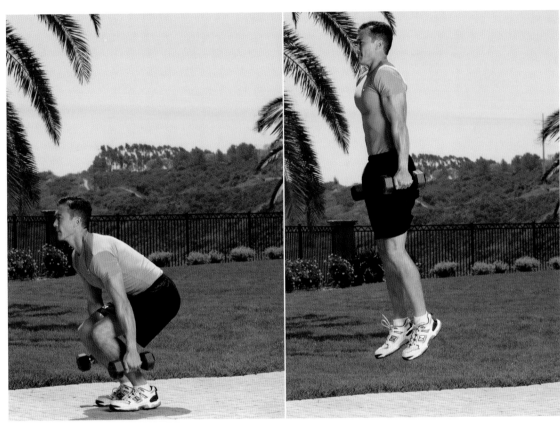

Dumbbell squat jumps; 30 reps (legs and cardio)

1. Start with your feet shoulder width apart and the DBs in your hands with your arms by your sides.

2. Begin the squat by pressing your hips back and bending your knees.

3. Propel yourself back up, jumping into the air.

4. Make sure when you land you land with soft knees.

5. Lower yourself back down and repeat the squat jump.

6. Maintain a neutral spine and control the DBs (don't let them swing).

7. Do a total of 30 reps, 15 on each side.

Repeat exercises 7–9, following your stage 2 calendar guidelines of sets and repetitions

exercise 10

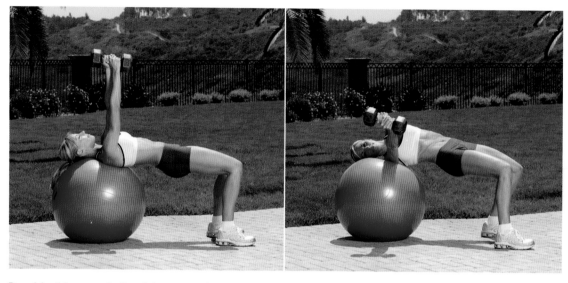

Dumbbell torso rotation lying on stability ball; 30 reps (abdominals and core)

1 Start by sitting on the ball, holding one DB in both hands.

2 Lean back slightly, engaging the abdominals, and slightly roll your body down into a bridge position on the ball while holding the DB in your hands extended straight over your shoulders to the ceiling.

3 Your head, neck, and upper back should be in contact with the ball at all times.

4 While keeping your arms straight, rotate the DB to your left side, bring it back to the middle, and then rotate it to the right side.

5 Repeat the rotation from side to side, squeezing your abdominals.

6 Do a total of 30 total reps, 15 on each side.

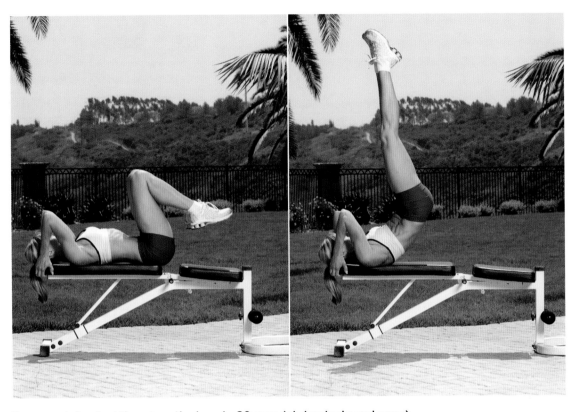

Reverse abdominal thrust on the bench; 30 reps (abdominals and arms)

1 Lie on your back on the bench, with your legs extended up and your feet pointing toward the ceiling.

2 Bring your arms up and over your head, grabbing the bench behind you.

3 Engaging your abs, pull your belly button in toward your spine, and lift or thrust your hips off the bench as high as you can, pushing your feet straight up.

4 Lower your hips slowly back toward the bench and repeat.

5 Do a total of 30 reps.

exercise 12

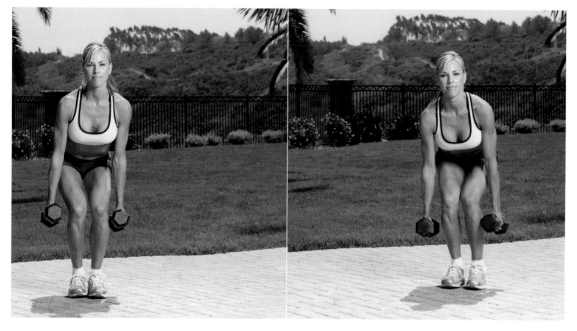

Ski jumps with dumbbells; 30 reps (legs and cardio)

1 With the DBs in your hands, stand with your feet together, bend your knees slightly, and press your hips back.

2 Keeping your feet together for the entire exercise, jump from side to side. Each jump should cover 6 to 18 inches.

3 Make sure your upper body stays upright and strong, and don't swing the DBs.

4 Do a total of 30 reps, 15 on each side.

Repeat exercises 10–12, following your stage 2 calendar guidelines of sets and repetitions

OKAY, NOW YOU'RE DONE WITH THE stage 2, day 1 resistance routine. Great job! Please make sure you stretch and drink plenty of water to stay hydrated. Follow your stage 2 workout calendar for your daily workout plan. Stay motivated and make the time you need to reach your goals. You are on your way to Ultrafitness!

Day 2: Shoulder, Biceps, Triceps, Core, and Cardio Intervals

EQUIPMENT NEEDED

- Hand weights or dumbbells (DB): I recommend an array of both light and heavier dumbbell weights to allow you to progress with the program and adjust the level of resistance in each exercise based on your level of fatigue. (Remember: Aim for an amount of weight that makes you fatigued in the last three reps.)
- Stability ball (55 cm is appropriate for most people): Inflate the ball so that when you are sitting on it, your knees are at a 90-degree angle.
- Floor space (with a mat or towel for comfort)
- Exercise bench or aerobic step
- Jump rope: When standing on the rope, the ends of the rope should end up directly under your armpits.

EXERCISE FORMAT

- All sets and repetitions (reps) are as stated on the stage 2 calendar (unless otherwise noted).
  Example: Week 1 = 2 sets of each exercise for 12 repetitions.
- The exercises are organized into super-sets: Complete each series of three before moving on to the next. For example: Week 6 = 3 sets of 15, 12, 10 repetitions (you'll do each super-set three times before moving on to the next).
- When the set repetitions are stated as a pyramid (e.g., 15, 12, 10), your corresponding weight should go up as the reps go down (e.g., 10 lbs., 12 lbs., 15 lbs.).
- When an exercise involves switching sides, complete a set on one side and then complete the same number of repetitions on the other side.
- Don't forget to refer to the illustrations in the book for proper form and movement.

exercise 1

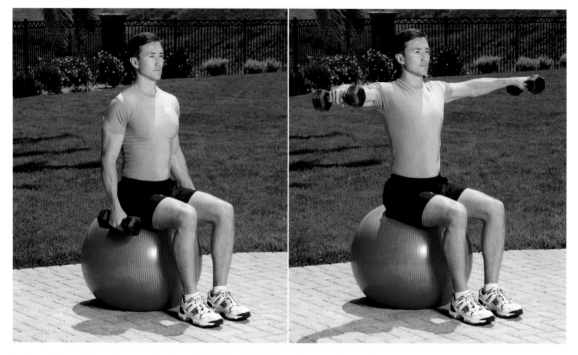

Lateral shoulder raise seated on stability ball (shoulders and core)

1	Sit on the ball with your torso tall and erect.
2	With the DBs down at your sides and your palms facing in, raise your arms out away from you.
3	Bring the DBs up only to shoulder height, and then lower back down; repeat.

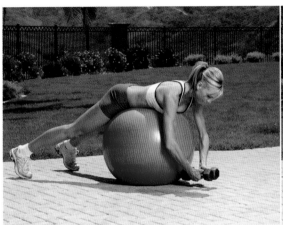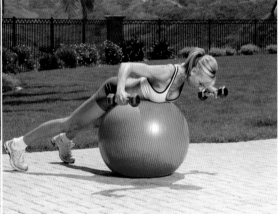

Rear deltoid raise bent over stability ball (shoulders and core)

1 Get on your knees with the DBs in your hands and bring the ball into contact with your torso; maintain contact throughout the exercise.

2 Bring yourself into a prone position by rolling yourself forward so you are on top of the ball.

3 Keep yourself in a neutral spine and keep your head and shoulders up (don't drop your head).

4 If your feet slide, secure them up against a wall or piece of furniture.

5 With your arms hanging by your sides and palms facing behind you, squeeze your shoulder blades together.

6 Draw your elbows out to your sides and up toward the ceiling.

7 Make sure your shoulder and elbow are in line with each other so you activate the rear deltoid.

8 Lower the DBs back down; repeat.

Jump rope for 2 minutes (cardio interval)

1 Make sure you have plenty of room and go for it.

2 Jump rope for 2 minutes as fast as you can.

Repeat exercises 1–3, following your stage 2 calendar guidelines of sets and repetitions

exercise 4

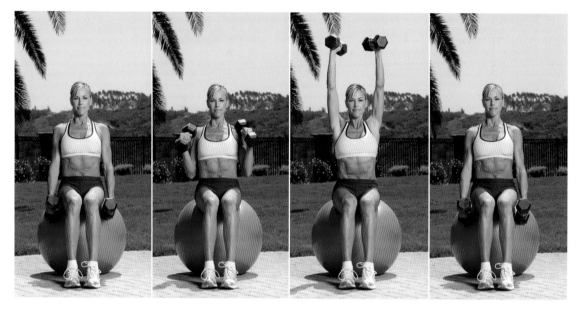

Hammer curl and shoulder press combo seated on stability ball (biceps, shoulders, and core)

1 Sit on the ball with the DBs in your hands and your arms at your sides, palms facing in.

2 Draw the DBs up to your shoulders for the biceps curl.

3 From the shoulder, press the DBs overhead, keeping your elbows pointing forward.

4 Bring the DBs back down to your shoulders and then lower the DBs back down to your sides by straightening your elbows; repeat, starting with the biceps curl.

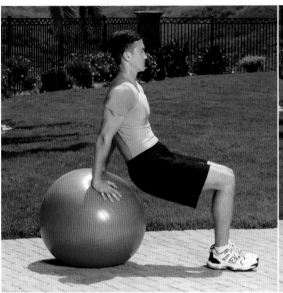 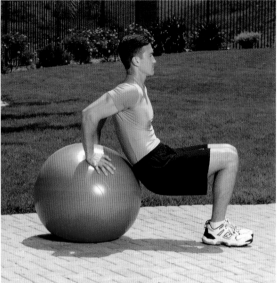

Triceps dip off the stability ball (triceps and balance)

1 Sit on the ball with your hands by your sides pressing into the ball and your fingertips facing forward.

2 Lift your hips off the ball and walk your feet out two steps.

3 Keep your shoulders away from your ears and your spine in neutral.

4 Bend your elbows, lowering your hips and keeping your weight in your hands on the ball.

5 Straighten your elbows back up; repeat.

Jump rope for 2 minutes (cardio interval)

1 Give it everything you've got for 2 minutes.

Repeat exercises 4–6, following your stage 2 calendar guidelines of sets and repetitions

exercises 7, 8, 9

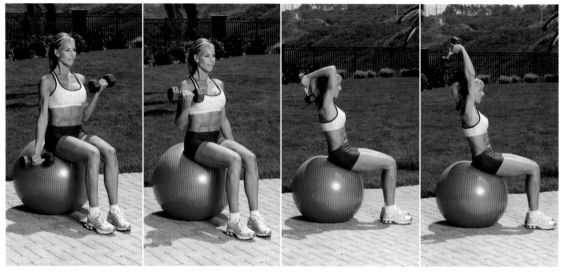

Alternating biceps curl seated on stability ball (biceps and core)

1	Sit on the ball with the DBs in your hands, palms facing forward.
2	Moving one arm at a time, raise the DB by bending your elbow and lift the DB to your shoulder.
3	Lower the DB back down slowly and repeat on the other side.

Triceps overhead extension seated on stability ball (triceps and core)

1	Sit on the ball with one DB in both hands over your head.
2	Bend both elbows and lower the DB behind your head toward the floor.
3	Extend your elbows back up, raising the DB back over your head.
4	Keep your abs tight and your spine straight.
5	Repeat.

Jump rope for 2 minutes (cardio interval)

1	Jump as fast as you can for 2 minutes.

Repeat exercises 7–9, following your stage 2 calendar guidelines of sets and repetitions.

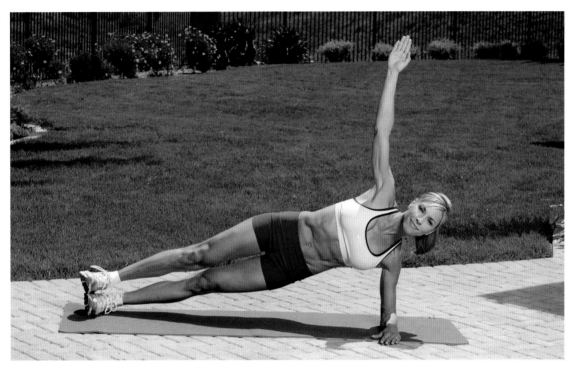

Side plank hold on elbow for 60 seconds (shoulders and core)

1 Lie on your right side, propped up on your right elbow with your knees bent in front of you.

2 Extend your top leg so that your body is straight from head to toe.

3 Leaning into the right forearm, lift up your hips and extend your bottom leg.

4 Make sure you don't drop into the shoulder; maintain shoulder girdle stability.

5 The 60-second hold doesn't begin until you're up in the plank.

6 Repeat the side plank on your left side for 60 seconds.

exercise 11

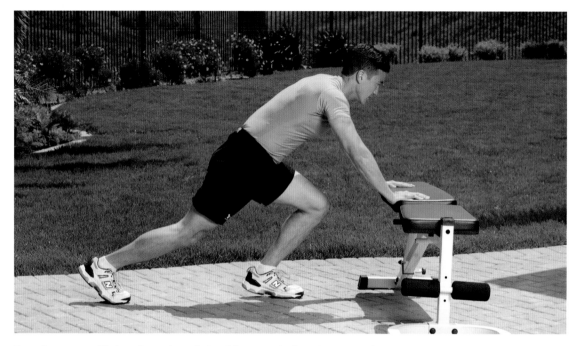

Running man with hands on bench for 60 seconds (cardio, upper body strength, and core)

1 Get on the floor with your hands on the bench and hold a push-up position with your toes down.

2 Make sure you keep your spine neutral and maintain shoulder girdle stability.

3 Bring your right knee into your chest.

4 Switch foot positions quickly, bringing your right leg back and your left knee into your chest.

5 Repeat as fast as you can for 60 seconds.

Repeat exercises 10 and 11, following your stage 2 calendar guidelines of sets and repetitions

YOU'RE NOW DONE WITH THE STAGE 2, day 2 resistance routine. How great do you feel about yourself now? Make sure you stretch and drink plenty of water to stay hydrated. Follow your stage 2 workout calendar for your daily workout plan. Keep yourself motivated by reviewing your goals and tracking your progress as you go. You are on your way to Ultrafitness!

Cardio Exercise Details

STAGE 2

Stage 2: Ultrafit Treadmill Blast!

This workout can be performed outside without a machine if you don't have access to a treadmill; you just have to increase your speed if the required incline is unavailable. Try to find a hilly area so you can walk that for the second part of the workout. I like to use a treadmill because you can adjust your pace and incline instantly to keep things exciting. Using your scale of perceived exertion (scaling effort from 1 to 10), you will need to determine for yourself what slow-, medium-, and fast-paced walking means to you. When you change speeds and/or inclines, make those transitions as quickly as possible.

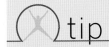

If the workout becomes too difficult for you, bring your effort level down until you are fully recovered and then jump right back into it. Remember to check your heart rate regularly and maintain the appropriate heart rate zone. (I recommend using a heart rate monitor.)

A. WARM-UP: 10 MINUTES			
TIME	FORMAT	PACE	INCLINE
1 Minute	Walk	Slow	Flat (0%)
1 Minute	Jog	Medium	Flat
1 Minute	Walk	Medium	Flat
1 Minute	Jog	Medium	Flat
1 Minute	Walk	Medium	Flat
1 Minute	Jog	Medium	Flat
1 Minute	Walk	Medium	Flat
1 Minute	Jog	Medium	Flat
1 Minute	Walk	Medium	Flat
1 Minute	Jog	Medium	Flat

B. WORKING HARD: 10 MINUTES

TIME	FORMAT	PACE	INCLINE
1 Minute	Side Shuffle	Medium	Flat (right leg leads)
1 Minute	Side Shuffle	Medium	Flat (left leg leads)
1 Minute	Walk	Medium	3–4%
1 Minute	Jog	Medium	3–4%
1 Minute	Side Shuffle	Medium	Flat (right leg leads)
1 Minute	Side Shuffle	Medium	Flat (left leg leads)
1 Minute	Walk	Medium	5–6%
1 Minute	Jog	Medium	5–6%
1 Minute	Side Shuffle	Medium	Flat (right leg leads)
1 Minute	Side Shuffle	Medium	Flat (left leg leads)

20-MINUTE MARK! If your workout ends here, cool down for 1 minute by walking slowly on a flat grade. You're done—now STRETCH!

C. WORKING HARDER: 10 MINUTES

TIME	FORMAT	PACE	INCLINE
1 Minute	Jog	Medium	3–4%
1 Minute	Run	Fast	3–4%
1 Minute	Jog	Medium	3–4%
1 Minute	Run	Fast	3–4%
1 Minute	Jog	Medium	3–4%
1 Minute	Run	Fast	3–4%
1 Minute	Jog	Medium	3–4%
1 Minute	Run	Fast	3–4%
1 Minute	Jog	Medium	3–4%
1 Minute	Run	Fast	3–4%

30-MINUTE MARK! If your workout ends here, cool down for 1 minute by walking slowly on a flat grade. You're done—now STRETCH!!

Stage 2:
Ultrafit Stair Challenge

This workout requires a long set of stairs (preferably outside) that are safe to run on. I recommend visiting a local school stadium to see what's available. You can also use a step mill if one is available at your gym.

A. WARM-UP: 5 MINUTES

Step up and down on 1 step, right leg leading (up, up, down, down), for 30 seconds.

Step up and down on 1 step, left leg leading (up, up, down, down), for 30 seconds.

Walk up every step and walk down.

Walk up every other step and walk down.

Walk up every step and walk down.

Walk up every other step and walk down.

Step up and down on 1 step, right leg leading (up, up, down, down), for 30 seconds.

Step up and down on 1 step, left leg leading (up, up, down, down), for 30 seconds.

B. WORKING HARD: 5 MINUTES

Walk up every step and walk down.

Walk up every other step and walk down.

Stationary squats for 60 seconds.

Run up every step and walk down.

Run up every other step and walk down.

Stationary alternating forward lunges for 60 seconds.

Run up every step and jog down.

Run up every other step and jog down.

C. WORKING HARDER: 5 MINUTES

Run up every other step and jog down.

Walk up every 3 steps and jog down.

Push-up hold (on hands and toes) for 30 seconds.

Run up every other step and jog down.

Walk up every 3 steps and jog down.

Push-up hold (on hands and toes) for 30 seconds.

Side walk (with right leg leading) up every other step and jog down.

Side walk (with left leg leading) up every other step and jog down.

On your right leg only, hop up 2 steps, walk up 4 steps, and repeat; jog down.

On your left leg only, hop up 2 steps, walk up 4 steps, and repeat; jog down.

Sprint (as fast as you can) up every step and then jog down.

Repeat segments to increase workout time.

ARE YOU DONE? Make sure you stretch your calves, shins, hamstrings, glutes, quads, and lower back.

Stage 2: Ultrafit Boot Camp

All you need to complete this workout is a good pair of sneakers and access to outside terrain (preferably on sand, grass, or a running track). Have fun!

A. WARM-UP: 5 MINUTES

Side shuffle (right leg leading) for 60 seconds.

Side shuffle (left leg leading) for 60 seconds.

Jog backward for 60 seconds.

Jog forward for 60 seconds.

Power walk for 60 seconds.

B. WORKING HARD: 5 MINUTES

Quick feet for 30 seconds.

Heel kicks for 30 seconds.

Sprint as fast as you can for 30 seconds.

Stop and drop! Complete as many push-ups (from your toes) as you can in 30 seconds.

Turn over! Complete as many triceps dips as you can in 30 seconds.

Quick feet for 30 seconds.

Heel kicks for 30 seconds.

Sprint as fast as you can for 30 seconds.

Slow it down! Forward walking lunges for the next 60 seconds.

C. WORKING HARDER: 5 MINUTES

Jog forward for 60 seconds.

Stop where you are! Complete as many jump squats as you can in 30 seconds.

Jog backward for 60 seconds.

Stop where you are! Complete as many jump squats as you can in 30 seconds.

Sprint as fast as you can for 30 seconds.

The end is near! Complete as many backward lunges as you can in 30 seconds.

Drop down! Hold a right side plank for 30 seconds (see resistance training exercises on page 67 for a photo of the plank position for core training).

Switch sides! Hold a left side plank for 30 seconds.

Repeat segments to increase workout time.

ARE YOU DONE? Make sure you cool down and stretch!

Stage 2: Ultrafit Extreme Jump Rope

This workout requires just a jump rope and you. The best part about this workout is how easily it travels with you—so no excuses!

A. WARM-UP: 5 MINUTES

Basic jump rope (single or double hop) for 60 seconds.

Side to side jump rope for 60 seconds.

Basic jump rope (single or double hop) for 60 seconds.

Side to side jump rope for 60 seconds.

Basic jump rope (single or double hop) for 60 seconds.

B. WORKING HARD: 5 MINUTES

High knees jump rope for 60 seconds.

On your right leg only, jump rope for 60 seconds.

High knees jump rope for 60 seconds.

On your left leg only, jump rope for 60 seconds.

Speed jump rope for 60 seconds.

C. WORKING HARDER: 5 MINUTES

Speed jump rope for 2 minutes.

Slow jump rope for 60 seconds.

Speed jump rope for 2 minutes.

Repeat segments to increase workout time.

ARE YOU DONE? Make sure you cool down and stretch!

Stage 2: Ultrafit Bike Workout

You will need a stationary bike or Spin Cycle to complete this workout. You'll need to use your scale of perceived exertion (scaling effort from 1 to 10) combined with adjusting the bike tension on a scale of 1 to 10 throughout the workout.

A. WARM-UP: 10 MINUTES			
TIME	**FORMAT**	**PACE**	**TENSION**
1 Minute	Seated Cycle	Slow	None
1 Minute	Seated Cycle	Medium	None
1 Minute	Seated Cycle	Fast	None
1 Minute	Seated Cycle	Slow	2%
1 Minute	Seated Cycle	Medium	2%
1 Minute	Seated Cycle	Fast	2%
1 Minute	Seated Cycle	Medium	2%
1 Minute	Climbing Cycle	Medium	2%
1 Minute	Seated Cycle	Medium	4%
1 Minute	Climbing Cycle	Medium	4%

B. WORKING HARD: 10 MINUTES			
TIME	**FORMAT**	**PACE**	**TENSION**
2 Minutes	Climbing Cycle	Medium	4%
1 Minute	Climbing Cycle	Fast	4%
2 Minutes	Climbing Cycle	Medium	6%
1 Minute	Climbing Cycle	Fast	6%
2 Minutes	Climbing Cycle	Medium	8%
1 Minute	Climbing Cycle	Fast	8%
1 Minute	Seated Cycle	Fast	None

20-MINUTE MARK! If your workout ends here, cool down for 1 minute by pedaling slowly with no tension. You're done—now STRETCH!!

C. WORKING HARDER: 10 MINUTES

TIME	FORMAT	PACE	TENSION
1 Minute	Seated Cycle	Medium	4%
1 Minute	Seated Cycle	Fast	4%
1 Minute	Climbing Cycle	Fast	6%
1 Minute	Seated Cycle	Medium	6%
1 Minute	Seated Cycle	Fast	6%
1 Minute	Climbing Cycle	Fast	8%
1 Minute	Seated Cycle	Medium	8%
1 Minute	Seated Cycle	Fast	8%
1 Minute	Climbing Cycle	Fast	10%

30-MINUTE MARK! If your workout ends here, cool down for 1 minute by pedaling slowly with no tension. You're done—now STRETCH!

Stage 2: Ultrafit Sprint Intervals

As with the Boot Camp Workout, all you need to complete this workout is a good pair of workout shoes and access to outside terrain (preferably on sand, grass, or a running track). Have fun!

A. WARM-UP: 5 MINUTES

Moderate jog for 2 minutes.
High knees for 30 seconds.
Moderate jog for 2 minutes.
Heel kicks for 30 seconds.

B. WORKING HARD: 5 MINUTES

Quick feet for 10 seconds into a 10-second sprint; jog back to start.

Quick feet for 10 seconds into a 20-second sprint; jog back to start.

Quick feet for 10 seconds into a 30-second sprint; jog back to start.

Power skips (reach high!) for 60 seconds.

Quick feet for 10 seconds into a 10-second sprint; jog back to start.

Quick feet for 10 seconds into a 20-second sprint; jog back to start.

Quick feet for 10 seconds into a 30-second sprint; jog back to start.

C. WORKING HARDER: 5 MINUTES

Slow 20 seconds / moderate 20 seconds / fast 20 seconds speed buildup for a total of 60 seconds.

Slow jog for 30 seconds.

Slow 20 / moderate 20 / fast 20 speed buildup for a total of 60 seconds.

Slow jog for 30 seconds.

Slow 20 / moderate 20 / fast 20 speed buildup for a total of 60 seconds.

Power skips (reach high!) for 60 seconds.

Repeat segments to increase workout time.

TIME TO COOL DOWN AND STRETCH!

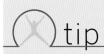

tip

It's extremely important that you breathe correctly and, at the same time, properly draw in your abdominal muscles prior to engaging in any of these exercises.

Ultrafit Core Training Details

You have a "corset" that wraps around your abdomen and back and is called the transverse abdominus, and once you learn to isolate the transverse abdominus, you'll be on your way to a stronger back and a flatter tummy. Imagine a string attached to the inside of your belly button. Take a deep breath through your nose and exhale through your mouth, while at the same time pulling the string toward your spine and drawing your belly button in. You should still be able to breathe correctly while holding this muscle in position.

EQUIPMENT NEEDED

- Hand weights
- Stability ball

EXERCISE FORMAT

- There are three super-sets of exercises (exercises to be performed back to back), each to be completed three times before moving on to the next super-set.

suggestions and definitions

This abdominal workout has been designed to target your entire "core" area. When I mention an "isometric" move (e.g., "V-sit isometric hold"), it actually refers to no movement at all. Isometric training requires you to sustain a muscle contraction over a given period of time, and there are no repetitions required.

The end result of isometric training is that the muscle begins to recruit and activate more motor units to help maintain this contraction, and the motor units are then forced to contract continuously, time after time, thus maturing the entire muscle very quickly.

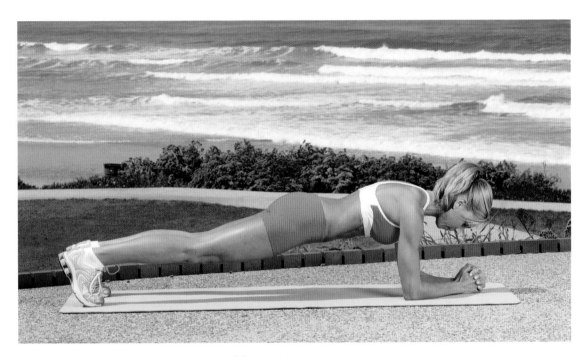

Plank hold from forearms and toes for 60 seconds

1	Get down on the floor on your hands and knees.
2	Bring yourself down so that you are resting on your forearms.
3	Make sure your shoulders are directly over your elbows and clasp your hands together.
4	Tighten up those abs and keep your spine long.
5	Extend both your legs so that your knees are off the ground and your toes are supporting you.
6	Your body should be straight from the tip of your head all the way through to your feet.
7	Make sure you don't drop into your shoulders or arch your back; maintain shoulder girdle stability.
8	The 60-second hold doesn't begin until you're up in the plank.

exercise 2

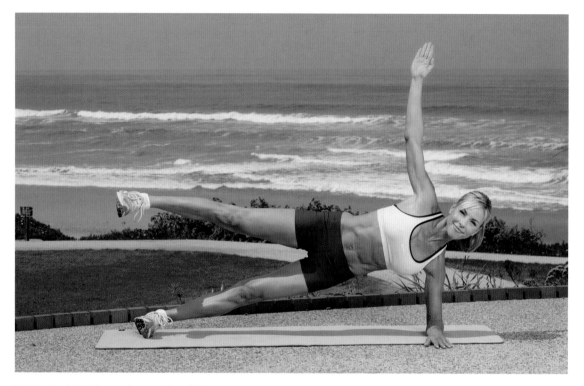

Side plank hold, one leg up, for 60 seconds

1. Bring yourself into the forearm plank hold as described earlier.

2. Bring your forearms together so they are touching, parallel to each other, and each hand is touching the opposite elbow.

3. Roll yourself onto your right elbow with your shoulder directly over the elbow.

4. You'll now be looking at the wall instead of the floor.

5. Make sure your hips are stacked on top of each other and your feet are stacked on top of each other.

6. Extend your left arm up to the ceiling, opening your chest, and at the same time lift your left leg up to increase the intensity.

7. Pull your abs in and breathe.

8. The 60-second hold doesn't begin until you're up in the plank on your right elbow with your left leg up.

9. Repeat the side plank on the left side for 60 seconds.

Repeat exercises 1 and 2 for 3 sets

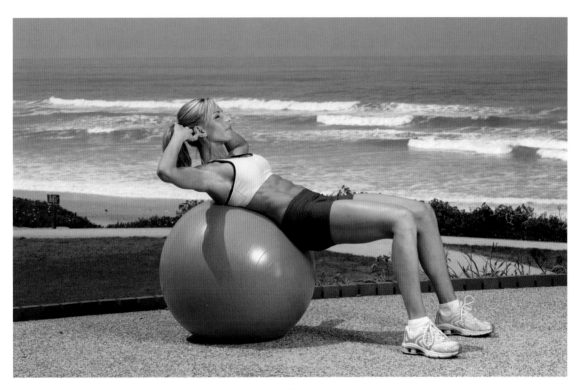

Abdominal crunches on stability ball, one leg up; 50 reps

1 Sit on the stability ball, tuck your pelvis, lean back, and walk your feet away from the ball.

2 Walk out until your lower back is supported on the stability ball and the tips of your shoulder blades are touching the ball.

3 Challenge: The more "on top" of the ball you are, the more difficult the exercise will be.

4 Bring your hands back so they are cradling your head; your eyes are on the ceiling and your elbows are open wide.

5 Pull in your abs as you lift your right leg so it is parallel to the floor.

6 Hold steady as you lift your torso up and pull your belly button toward your spine.

7 Lower your shoulders back down and do 25 reps with the right leg up and then 25 with the left leg up.

8 Don't let the stability ball move during the exercise.

exercise 4

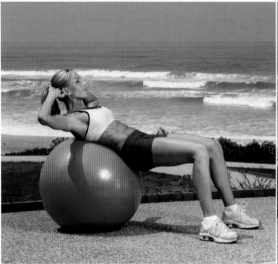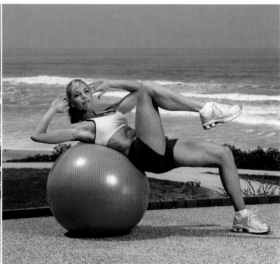

Alternating oblique crunches lying on stability ball; 50 reps

1 Sit on the stability ball, tuck your pelvis, lean back, and walk your feet away from the ball.

2 Walk out until your lower back is supported on the stability ball and the tips of your shoulder blades are touching the ball.

3 Challenge: The more "on top" of the ball you are, the more difficult the exercise will be.

4 Bring your hands back so they are cradling your head; your eyes are on the ceiling and your elbows are open wide.

5 Pull in your abs as you lift your left shoulder and bring your left elbow toward your right knee.

6 Bring your body back to center and repeat on the other side, alternating sides for 25 reps on each side.

7 Make sure the stability ball does not move during the exercise.

Repeat exercises 3 and 4 for 3 sets

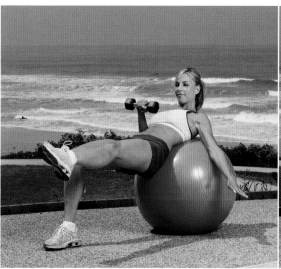 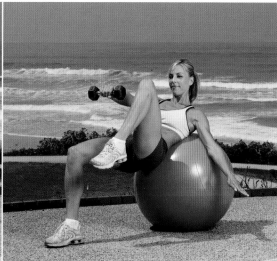

Dumbbell oblique punches lying on stability ball; 50 reps

1. Sit on the stability ball, tuck your pelvis, lean back, and walk your feet away from the ball.

2. Walk out until your lower back is supported on the stability ball and the tips of your shoulder blades are touching the ball.

3. Challenge: The more "on top" of the ball you are, the more difficult the exercise will be.

4. Hold one DB in your right hand by your chest and lift your left leg out straight in front of you; this is your starting position.

5. Rotate and lift your torso while punching the DB to your left knee, then come back to center, bringing the DB back to your chest.

6. Perform 25 reps on this side and then switch sides.

7. Make sure the stability ball does not move during the exercise.

Repeat exercises 3 through 5 for 3 sets

> GREAT JOB! NOW REMEMBER TO STRETCH.
> **Lying on the ball with your arms stretched out to your sides and your feet planted on the floor is a great way to stretch out your abdominal area.**

stage 3 ultrafit program

Welcome to the stage 3, 6-week Ultrafit program! If you have already finished the stage 1 and 2 programs, then congratulations! If you have skipped the stage 1 and 2 programs and are starting with the stage 3 program, then I want to encourage you for beginning your new path to Ultrafitness! This stage is the most difficult stage in my book.

The calendar on pages 114–115 gives a brief overview of the workouts you will be doing for the next 6 weeks. Just as in the stage 1 and 2 programs, I did not get into exercise details on this calendar. All the details and pictures of the exercises will follow in this chapter. You will also notice my nutritional advice and goals to follow. If you have already finished the stage 1 and 2 programs, I would like you to begin again as you did 12 weeks ago and re-sign the pledge and follow the stage 3 nutritional advice like before. If this is new to you, then here's how to follow the calendar.

For each day, I give a suggested amount of water for you to drink. This is only a suggestion and you can decide for yourself whether this is the right amount for you. I am only trying to get you to increase your water intake each day, but you should never exceed a gallon, or 128 ounces. Begin with Monday as day 1. For this first day, you will need to do Weights D1 2 x 12 reps.

D1 stands for day 1 of the resistance training workouts I have prepared for you, and 2 x 12 reps means you are to do 2 sets of 12 repetitions of each exercise unless otherwise noted on the workout. Some exercises require you to do more repetitions. It also tells you to do the 30-minute Extreme Jump Rope workout. You will find this workout explained in the cardio section.

I have planned two resistance-training days, day 1 and day 2. Day 1 consists of chest, back, legs, and core training. I have also added plyometric training (or higher intensity workouts) to step up your fitness and to push you to your max! Day 2 you will be working your shoulders, biceps, triceps, and core. Also in day 2, I have added cardio intervals to increase your heart rate with interval training and help you burn the maximum amount of calories. The calendar will tell you which one to do and on which day.

I have designed the workouts this way to give you a variety of different strength-training exercises to improve strength and body leanness. I always add in core training, so you will be working your abdominals without even knowing it and will improve your core strength, giving you ideal functional strength to prepare you for real-life situations that require total body power. The cardio workouts provide you with a cross-training program that will not only push you to your limit but also give you enough variety so you won't get bored. I use intervals throughout the strength training and cardio workouts to help you burn more calories and increase your cardiovascular endurance and health.

You will also notice as you progress through the 6 weeks that I have increased your sets, reps, and amount of cardio that I expect you to do. This is simply because you should be getting stronger and more cardiovascularly fit as the weeks go on. You are the judge for yourself. I try to push you, but only you know whether you are ready to progress. Remember, this is stage 3; you should be ready for these advanced workouts. If not, you might go back to stage 2 and repeat that 6 weeks until it becomes easier for you. Then you will know you are ready for stage 3.

If this stage 3 program becomes too easy for you, there are a few things you can do. You can increase the cardio workouts by repeating the third section (the most difficult); you can add weight in the strength-training sections; or you can increase the amount of plyometric (or high-intensity) training intervals in the day 1 strength-training workout or increase the cardio time in the day 2 strength-training workout. You could also play with the amount of reps and weight you do; for example, to decrease your pyramid training you could do 3 sets of 12, 10, and 8 reps and increase the weight, instead of doing 3 sets of 15, 12, and 10 reps at a lower weight. The idea is to push yourself and constantly change what you are doing so your body doesn't get used to the same old exercises all the time and hit a plateau.

I have also included an extra core-training workout and a stretch series. You are to do all of the workouts that are written on any given day. Also try to follow the times I have stated for each workout. You will notice that the amount of time for these cardio workouts will also increase as the weeks go by. If you can't do everything because of time or ability, don't beat yourself up.

Do what you can. This brings me to my next point: What to do if you don't have time one day to complete the entire workout. I tell my advanced clients to make time! If you want to take your body to the next level of Ultrafitness, then you need to be disciplined and strive for excellence. Make an appointment with yourself and this book every day for the entire 6 weeks and you won't be sorry!

Okay, so that is a little extreme and I am a workout freak, or so I've been told. If you truly don't have time one day, then I suggest doing either fewer reps than the suggested amount on the calendar or shortening the cardio section. You could skip one or the other, too. If I had my choice, I would do the strength training instead of the cardio section because the more muscle you have the higher your metabolism will be, thus your body will naturally burn more calories. You will be a fat-burning machine, and who doesn't want that? You don't want to do that all the time, though, because cardio is important, too. You can do this! Remember, you can do anything for 6 weeks.

calendar

	GOALS	MON	TUES	WED	THURS	FRI	SAT	SUN
WEEK 1	■ Sign pledge ■ Schedule checkup (if you have not already done so in stage 2) ■ Start food log ■ Start essential oil and supplements (see chapter 8) ■ Clean out cabinets/go grocery shopping ■ Write down five short-term and five long-term goals	☐ Weights D1 ☐ 2 x 12 Reps ☐ 30m Extreme Jump Rope ☐ 128 oz. H_2O	☐ Weights D2 ☐ 2 x 12 Reps ☐ 30m Bike Workout ☐ 128 oz. H_2O	☐ 30m Stair Challenge ☐ Core Training ☐ Stretch Series ☐ 128 oz. H_2O	☐ Weights D1 ☐ 2 x 12 Reps ☐ 30m Treadmill Blast! ☐ 128 oz. H_2O	☐ Weights D2 ☐ 2 x 12 Reps ☐ 30m Boot Camp ☐ 128 oz. H_2O	☐ 30m Sprint Intervals ☐ Core Training ☐ Stretch Series ☐ 128 oz. H_2O	☐ OFF ☐ 128 oz. H_2O
WEEK 2	■ No candy/junk food this week ■ No fast food this week ■ Make sure you're eating 5 to 6 small meals/day	☐ Weights D1 ☐ 3 x 12 Reps ☐ 30m Treadmill Blast! ☐ 128 oz. H_2O	☐ Weights D2 ☐ 3 x 12 Reps ☐ 30m Boot Camp ☐ 128 oz. H_2O	☐ 30m Sprint Intervals ☐ Core Training ☐ Stretch Series ☐ 128 oz. H_2O	☐ Weights D1 ☐ 3 x 12 Reps ☐ 30m Extreme Jump Rope ☐ 128 oz. H_2O	☐ Weights D2 ☐ 3 x 12 Reps ☐ 30m Bike Workout ☐ 128 oz. H_2O	☐ 30m Stair Challenge ☐ Core Training ☐ Stretch Series ☐ 128 oz. H_2O	☐ OFF ☐ 128 oz. H_2O
WEEK 3	■ Write down five things you like about your body ■ Exercise in the morning before breakfast this week ■ Cut out high-fat condiments and dairy	☐ Weights D1 ☐ 3 x 15 Reps ☐ 20m Treadmill Blast! ☐ 20m Extreme Jump Rope ☐ 128 oz. H_2O	☐ Weights D2 ☐ 3 x 15 Reps ☐ 20m Bike Workout ☐ 20m Boot Camp ☐ 128 oz. H_2O	☐ 30m Stair Challenge ☐ Core Training ☐ Stretch Series ☐ 128 oz. H_2O	☐ Weights D1 ☐ 3 x 15 Reps ☐ 20m Treadmill Blast! ☐ 20m Extreme Jump Rope ☐ 128 oz. H_2O	☐ Weights D2 ☐ 3 x 15 Reps ☐ 20m Bike Workout ☐ 20m Boot Camp ☐ 128 oz. H_2O	☐ 30m Sprint Intervals ☐ Core Training ☐ Stretch Series ☐ 128 oz. H_2O	☐ OFF ☐ 128 oz. H_2O

	GOALS	MON	TUES	WED	THURS	FRI	SAT	SUN
WEEK 4	■ No alcohol for the next three weeks ■ Go to bed 1 hour earlier three times this week ■ Make sure you're getting 25 to 30g of fiber/day	☐ Weights D1 ☐ 3 x 15, 12, 10 ☐ 20m Treadmill Blast! ☐ 20m Extreme Jump Rope ☐ 128 oz. H_2O	☐ Weights D2 ☐ 3 x 15, 12, 10 ☐ 20m Bike Workout ☐ 20m Boot Camp ☐ 128 oz. H_2O	☐ 40m Sprint Intervals ☐ Core Training ☐ Stretch Series ☐ 128 oz. H_2O	☐ Weights D1 ☐ 3 x 15, 12, 10 ☐ 20m Treadmill Blast! ☐ 20m Extreme Jump Rope ☐ 128 oz. H_2O	☐ Weights D2 ☐ 3 x 15, 12, 10 ☐ 20m Bike Workout ☐ 20m Boot Camp ☐ 128 oz. H_2O	☐ 40m Stair Challenge ☐ Core Training ☐ Stretch Series ☐ 128 oz. H_2O	☐ OFF ☐ 128 oz. H_2O
WEEK 5	■ Make two new healthy recipes this week ■ Write down five affirmations	☐ Weights D1 ☐ 3 x 12, 10, 8 ☐ 20m Treadmill Blast! ☐ 30m Extreme Jump Rope ☐ 128 oz. H_2O	☐ Weights D2 ☐ 3 x 12, 10, 8 ☐ 20m Bike Workout ☐ 30m Boot Camp ☐ 128 oz. H_2O	☐ 40m Stair Challenge ☐ Core Training ☐ Stretch Series ☐ 128 oz. H2O	☐ Weights D1 ☐ 3 x 12, 10, 8 ☐ 30m Treadmill Blast! ☐ 20m Extreme Jump Rope ☐ 128 oz. H_2O	☐ Weights D2 ☐ 3 x 12, 10, 8 ☐ 30m Bike Workout ☐ 20m Boot Camp ☐ 128 oz. H_2O	☐ 40m Sprint Intervals ☐ Core Training ☐ Stretch Series ☐ 128 oz. H_2O	☐ OFF ☐ 128 oz. H_2O
WEEK 6	■ Review your short-term and long-term goals ■ Treat yourself to some new piece of clothing	☐ Weights D1 ☐ 3 x 20 Reps ☐ 20m Treadmill Blast! ☐ 30m Extreme Jump Rope ☐ 128 oz. H_2O	☐ Weights D2 ☐ 3 x 20 Reps ☐ 20m Bike Workout ☐ 30m Boot Camp ☐ 128 oz. H_2O	☐ 40m Sprint Intervals ☐ Core Training ☐ Stretch Series ☐ 128 oz. H_2O	☐ Weights D1 ☐ 3 x 20 Reps ☐ 30m Treadmill Blast! ☐ 20m Extreme Jump Rope ☐ 128 oz. H_2O	☐ Weights D2 ☐ 3 x 20 Reps ☐ 30m Bike Workout ☐ 20m Boot Camp ☐ 128 oz. H_2O	☐ 40m Stair Challenge ☐ Stretch Series ☐ 128 oz. H_2O	☐ OFF ☐ 128 oz. H_2O

suggestions & definitions

- When selecting a set of dumbbells for your stage 3 workout, it should be very hard to complete the recommended number of reps for each exercise.
- When breathing through the exercises, exhale on the concentric (the contraction) movement and inhale on the eccentric (the release).
- When I refer to a "neutral spine," I am referring to the position of the spine. Your pelvis is not tilted, your neck is long, your abs are tight, and you are looking long and stable.
- When I refer to "shoulder girdle stability," I am referring to stabilizing your shoulder area by engaging or squeezing the shoulder blades and maintaining a strong upper body.

STAGE 3 Resistance Exercise Details

Day 1: Chest, Back, Legs, and Abdominals

EQUIPMENT NEEDED

- Hand weights or dumbbells (DB): I recommend an array of both light and heavier dumbbell weights to allow you to progress with the program and adjust the level of resistance in each exercise based on your level of fatigue. (Remember: Aim for an amount of weight that makes you fatigued in the last three sets.)
- Stability ball (55 cm is appropriate for most people): Inflate the ball so when you are sitting on it, your knees are at a 90-degree angle.
- Floor space (with a mat or towel for comfort)
- Exercise bench or aerobic step
- Jump rope: When standing on the rope, the ends of the rope should end up directly under your armpits.

EXERCISE FORMAT

- All sets and repetitions (reps) are as stated on the Stage 3 Calendar (unless otherwise stated)
- Don't forget to refer to the illustrations in the book for proper form and movement.

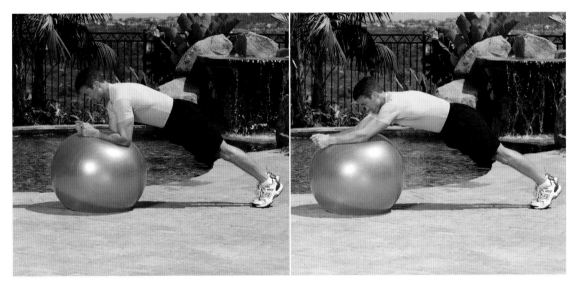

Straight arm lat roll with stability ball (back and core)

1 Get on your knees with your hands on the ball, and start with the ball arm's length away.

2 Keep your arms straight. You can stay on your knees or go to your toes to make the movement more advanced. Roll the ball as far away from you as you can while maintaining a neutral spine and shoulder girdle stability.

3 Engage the "lats" (side of your back) as you push into the ball; with straight arms, roll the ball back to the starting position.

4 Repeat.

exercise 2

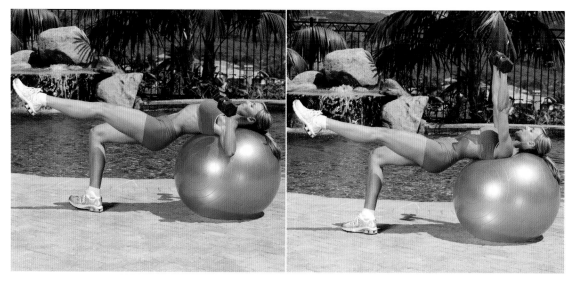

Dumbbell chest press from one-legged stability ball bridge (chest and core)

1. Holding both DBs, sit on the ball and rest the DBs on your thighs.

2. Tuck your pelvis, lean back, and walk your feet away from the ball.

3. Keep the ball in contact with your spine at all times as you roll out.

4. The bridge is complete when your head and shoulders are supported on the ball.

5. Challenge: As you lift your hips higher in the bridge, the exercise gets more difficult.

6. Bring the DBs from your thighs and take them over your shoulders and up to the ceiling.

7. Keep your hips in the starting position, and maintain a strong neutral spine throughout the exercise.

8. While maintaining the bridge, extend one leg out and hold.

9. Lower both DBs toward your shoulders by drawing your elbows out to the sides and down.

10. Press both DBs back up to the ceiling and stabilize your position; repeat.

11. Complete the same number of reps with the right leg up as you did with the left leg up.

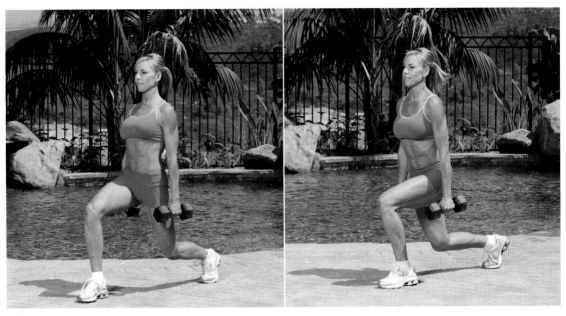

Plyometric lunge jumps with dumbbells (legs and cardio)

1 Start with a split stance position and the DBs in your hands.

2 Stand on your left leg, with your right leg extended behind you and your back heel up.

3 Your upper body should be in control with your hands on your hips.

4 Bend both knees and press your hips back slightly.

5 Jump and switch leg positions, with the right leg in front and the left leg in back.

6 Bend your knees again and repeat.

7 Make sure you don't swing the weights.

8 Do a total of 30 reps—15 on each side.

Repeat exercises 1–3, following your stage 3 calendar guidelines of sets and repetitions

exercise 4

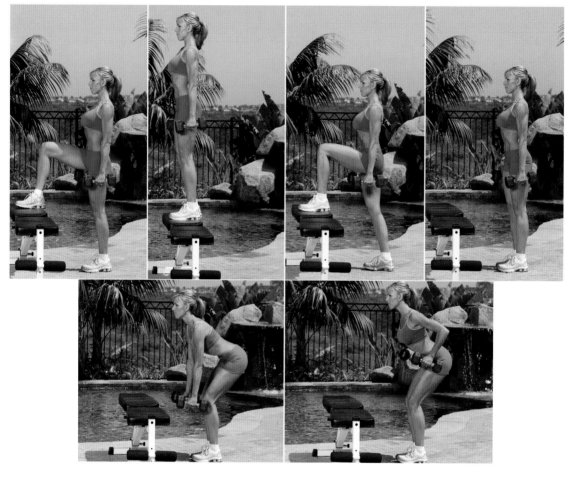

Step-ups and dumbbell back row combo (cardio, legs, and back)

1 Holding a DB in each hand, step up onto your bench with your right leg leading, and then step down.

2 Move right into a bent over two arm row.

3 When bending over, keep your spine straight, your knees soft, and your abs tight.

4 When rowing, squeeze your shoulder blades first and then draw your elbows up to your sides and lower back down.

5 Stand back up and repeat the entire exercise with the left leg leading.

6 Complete the same number of reps on each leg.

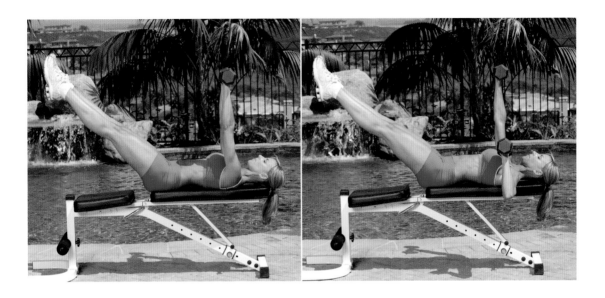

Alternating dumbbell chest press on bench with legs at 45 degrees (chest and core)

1 Lie on your bench with the DBs in your hands and your arms straight over your shoulders.

2 Bring your knees into your chest and then extend your legs straight up into the air.

3 Challenge: Engage those abs and lower your legs to a 45-degree angle; hold that position.

4 Begin the chest press by lowering one DB at a time and pressing it back up.

5 Repeat on the other side.

exercise 6

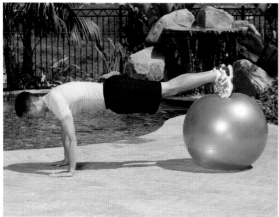 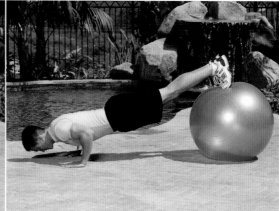

Decline push-ups off stability ball (chest and core)

1. Get on your knees with the ball in front of you.

2. Roll yourself over the ball and then begin to walk your hands out and away.

3. You will walk yourself out into a push-up position with a neutral spine; keep your abs tight and maintain shoulder girdle stability.

4. Challenge: The farther out you walk your hands, the harder the exercise will be.

5. Find a position you can maintain and hold it with your hands shoulder width apart.

6. Begin your push-up by bending your elbows out to the sides and lowering your torso.

7. Keeping your weight in your hands, press yourself back up; repeat.

8. Don't let the ball move during the exercise.

Repeat exercises 4–6, following your stage 3 calendar guidelines of sets and repetitions

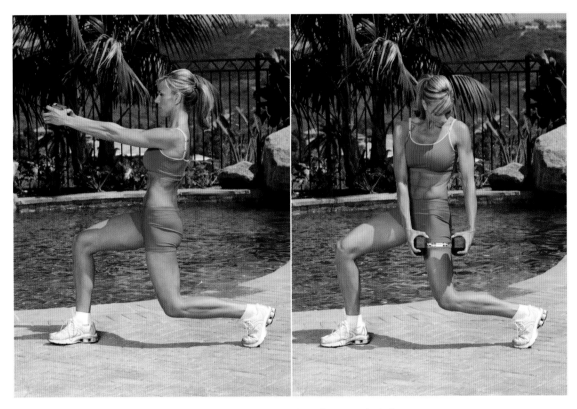

Alternating reverse lunge with dumbbell torso rotation (legs and abs)

1. Standing with your feet together, hold one DB with both hands in front of your thighs.

2. While stepping back with your right leg into a reverse lunge and keeping your back heel off the ground, raise your arms, holding the DB straight in front of you; as you step back, lower your body by bending your knees.

3. Holding that position, keep your abs tight as you rotate your torso and the DB to the right, toward your right foot.

4. Rotate your torso and DB back to the front and bring your right leg back together with the left.

5. Repeat the entire exercise with the left leg behind you and rotating to the left.

6. Stay balanced and upright with strong posture.

exercise 8

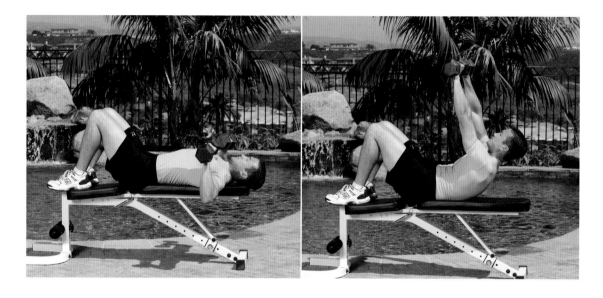

Dumbbell chest press with abdominal crunch (chest and abdominals)

1 Lie on your bench with the DBs in your hands and your arms extended over your shoulders.

2 Lower the DBs down toward your shoulders by bending your elbows.

3 Keep your abs tight and your lower back secure.

4 As you press the DBs back up, lift your head and shoulders up and crunch.

5 As you lower your head and shoulders back down, begin to lower the DBs again.

6 Repeat the chest press and crunch.

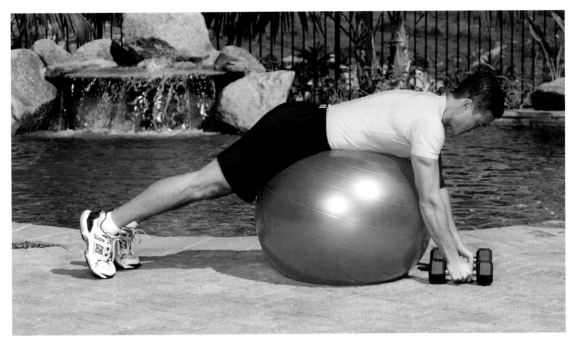

Dumbbell row on stability ball (back and core)

1 Start on your knees with the ball in front of you and the DBs in front of the ball. Slowly roll onto the ball, keeping your toes on the ground. Grab the DBs.

2 Holding this position and starting with your right arm, do a one-arm row. Keep your elbow close to your body, bring it up toward your back, squeeze and bring the DB back to the ground

3 Maintain tight abs and keep your neck in a neutral position.

4 Repeat this exercise with the right arm to complete the number of reps and then switch to your left arm.

Repeat exercises 7–9, following your stage 3 calendar guidelines of sets and repetitions

exercise 10

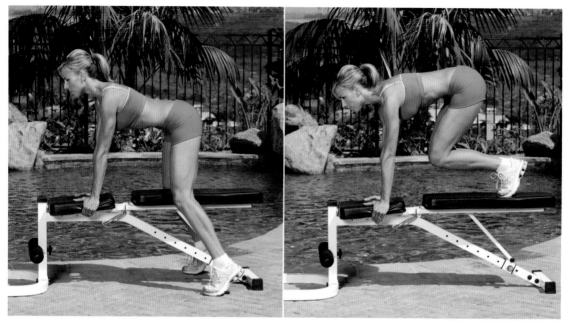

Straddle jump-ups for 1 minute (legs and cardio)

1 Stand straddling the bench; bend your knees and place your hands comfortably at the front on the bench.

2 Drop your hips, jump off the ground, and bring your feet onto the bench while keeping your hands on the bench.

3 Keeping your hands on the bench, jump up and place your feet back onto the ground and return to the starting position.

4 Do these straddle jump-ups for 1 minute.

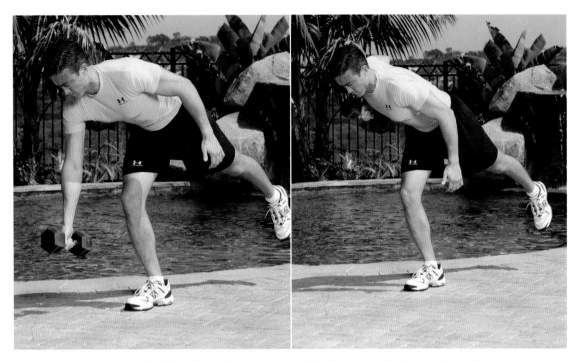

Stationary reaching single dead lift and one arm dumbbell row (back, legs, and core)

1. Start by standing on your right leg with a DB in your right hand.

2. Reach your body forward from your right arm; reach the DB toward the ground in front by lowering your body and extending your left leg out behind you.

3. Hold the position, balancing and keeping your back straight.

4. From this position, squeeze your back and do a one arm DB row with your right arm.

5. Lower the DB back down and slowly stand back up.

6. Do the same number of reps on the left side.

exercise 12

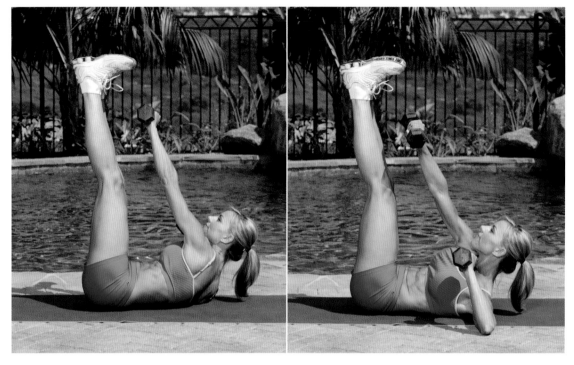

Abdominal dumbbell cross punch with feet in air (abdominals)

1 Lie on your back with the DBs in your hands and your legs straight up in the air.

2 Start with the DBs by your shoulders and your head and shoulders hovering off the ground, abs tight.

3 As you begin your crunch, reach the left DB toward your right foot, then lower yourself and the DB back down.

4 Crunch again and reach the right DB toward your left foot.

5 Alternate sides.

Repeat exercises 10–12, following your stage 3 calendar guidelines of sets and repetitions.

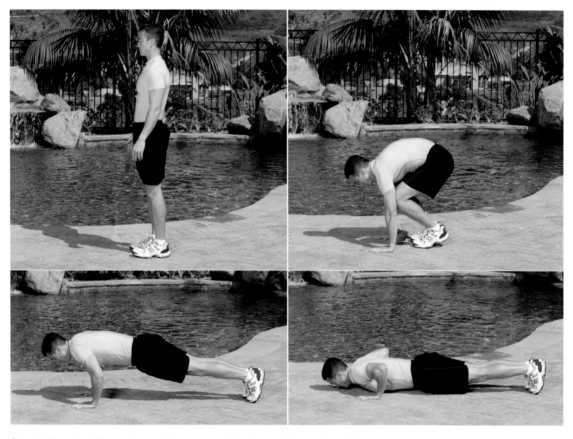

Squat thrust with push-ups (legs, upper body, cardio, and core)

1 Squat down, bringing your hands to the floor.

2 With your hands down, jump your feet back so you are in a push-up position.

3 Do 1 push-up.

4 Jump your feet back up to your hands and stand back up; repeat.

5 Maintain a strong upper body throughout the entire exercise.

exercise 14

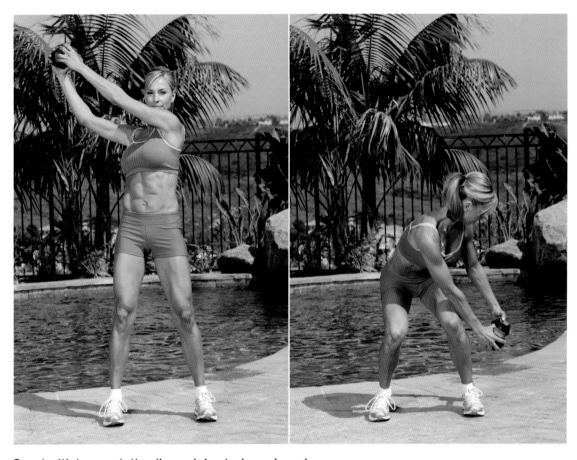

Squat with torso rotation (legs, abdominals, and core)

1 Keep your feet slightly wider than shoulder width apart; take one DB in both hands and hold it up over your head and to the right side.

2 Squat down and rotate your torso to the left while lowering the DB toward the floor and your left foot.

3 Stand back up, rotating the DB back to your starting position over your right shoulder. Repeat.

4 Switch sides and repeat.

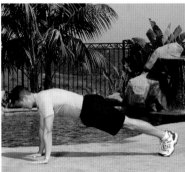 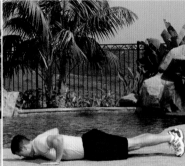 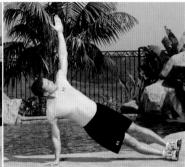

Push-ups with alternating side oblique rotation (chest, abdominals, and core)

1   Get into a push-up position with your hands close and your legs wide apart; do 1 push-up.

2   From the top of the push-up, rotate your torso and left arm out laterally; reach for the ceiling and look up.

3   Lower your left hand back to the floor and begin again by doing another push-up; reach up and twist to the right side.

4   Keep your abs in tight.

5   Challenge: You can do this exercise with light weights in your hands for added resistance.

Repeat exercises 13–15, following your stage 3 calendar guidelines of sets and repetitions

YOU'RE NOW DONE WITH THE STAGE 3, day 1 resistance routine. Great job! Please make sure you stretch and drink plenty of water to stay hydrated. Follow your stage 3 workout calendar for your daily workout plan. This is a tough workout, so be proud of yourself!

exercise 1

Day 2: Shoulders, Biceps, Triceps, Core, and Cardio Intervals

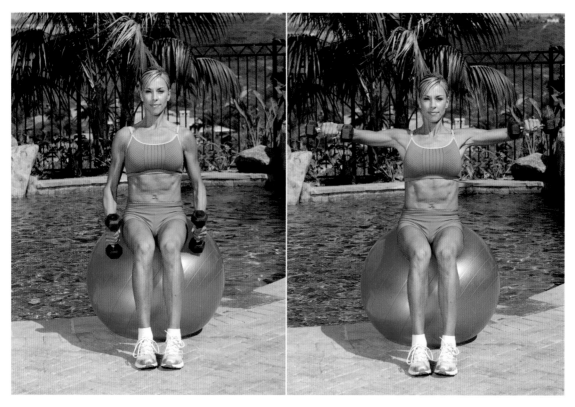

Lateral raise drop sets seated on stability ball (shoulders and core)

1 Have three sets of weights ready, with the heaviest being a weight with which you could do 10 reps of side lateral raises, though it would be difficult. The next two weight sizes should be slightly lighter. Example: 12lbs., 10lbs., and 8lbs.

2 Sitting on the ball, grab your heaviest set of DBs.

3 Sitting tall, raise your arms out to the sides and lift them up, keeping your elbows soft, then lower the DBs back down. Do 10 reps.

4 Drop that weight and pick up the middle weight; repeat the exercise for 10 reps.

5 Drop that weight, pick up the lightest weight, and repeat the exercise for 10 reps.

6 Do all 30 reps with no breaks.

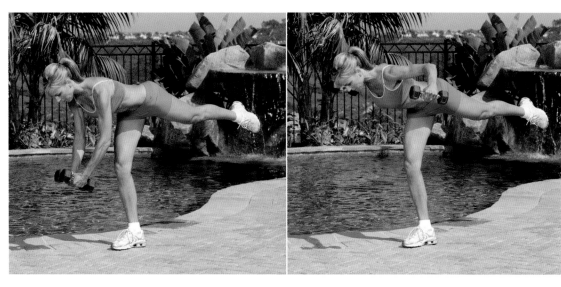

Single leg scale balance with rear deltoid raise (rear deltoid and core)

1 Balance on your left leg with the DBs in your hands.

2 Bring your torso toward the floor, balancing on your left leg, and extend your right leg behind you so your body is almost parallel to the floor; hold the DBs hanging down toward the floor.

3 Keeping your abs tight, perform rear deltoid raises by bringing the DBs out laterally to shoulder height and keeping a slight bend in your elbows. Squeeze the back of your shoulders and then return the DBs back down to the hanging position.

4 Stay in that balancing position until you finish your reps on that side.

5 Stand up slowly and repeat the exercise standing on your right leg. Repeat the same number of reps on each side.

Jump rope for 3 minutes (cardio interval)

1 Jump rope as fast as you can for 3 minutes.

Repeat exercises 1–3, following your stage 3 calendar guidelines of sets and repetitions

exercise 4

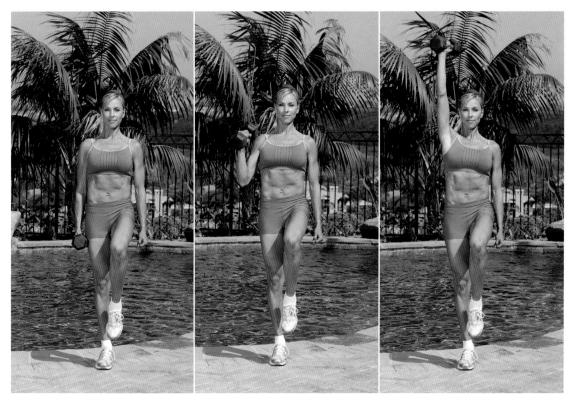

Single arm biceps curl into shoulder press combo standing on one leg (biceps, shoulders, and core)

1 Standing on your left leg, hold a DB in your right hand with your palm facing inward.

2 Maintaining your balance, bend your right elbow and bring the DB to your shoulder by squeezing your biceps.

3 From this position, press the DB overhead to a single arm shoulder press.

4 Lower the DB slowly back down to your starting position and repeat the combo.

5 Repeat the combo standing on your right leg with the DB in your left hand.

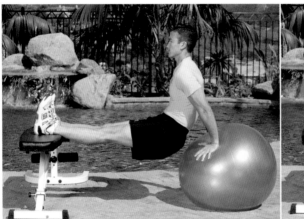 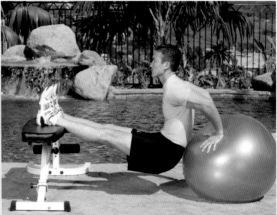

Triceps dip off the stability ball with feet elevated (triceps and core)

1 Sit on the ball with your hands by your sides pressing into the ball and your fingertips facing forward.

2 Lift your hips off the ball and walk your feet out 2 steps.

3 Bring your feet up onto your exercise bench.

4 Keep your shoulders away from your ears and your spine in neutral; stabilize your position.

5 Bend your elbows, lowering your hips and keeping your weight in your hands on the ball.

6 Straighten your elbows back up; repeat.

7 **NOTE:** If this too difficult with your feet elevated, put your feet on the floor.

Jump rope side to side for 3 minutes (cardio interval)

1 Jump rope with your feet together from side to side.

2 Go nice and fast for 3 minutes.

Repeat exercises 4–6, following your stage 3 calendar guidelines of sets and repetitions

exercise 7

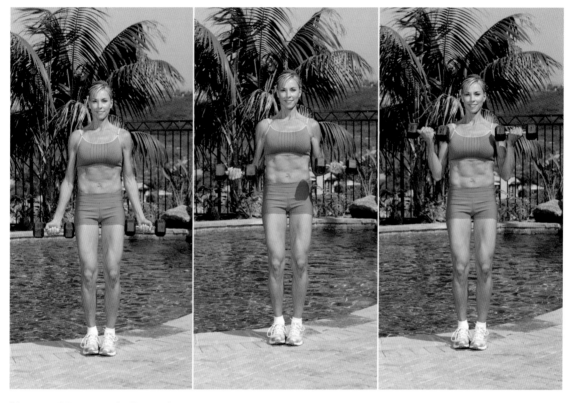

21-count biceps curls (biceps)

1 Stand with the DBs in your hands and your feet together.

2 Bending your elbows, lift the DBs from your sides to a 90-degree angle; do 7 reps.

3 Holding your elbows at 90 degrees, do 7 reps from 90 degrees up to your shoulders.

4 Do 7 more reps through the entire range of motion.

5 Do all 21 reps without stopping.

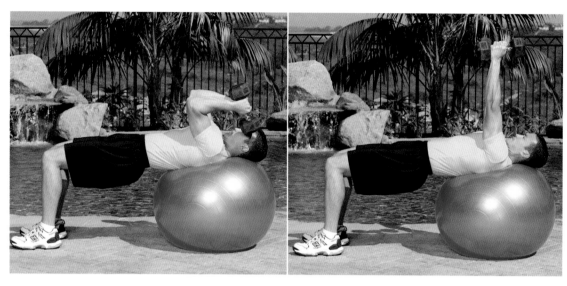

Stability ball bridge with triceps skull crusher (chest with balance challenge)

1. Holding both DBs, sit on the ball and rest the DBs on your thighs.

2. Tuck your pelvis, lean back, and walk your feet away from the ball, keeping the ball in contact with your spine at all times as your roll out.

3. The bridge is complete when your head and shoulders are supported on the ball.

4. Challenge: As you lift your hips higher in the bridge, the exercise gets more difficult.

5. Bring the DBs from your thighs and take them over your shoulders up to the ceiling.

6. Keep your hips in the starting position and maintain a strong neutral spine throughout the exercise.

7. Keeping your elbows over your shoulders, bend your elbows only and lower the DBs toward your head.

8. Keep your shoulders nice and stable and concentrate on your triceps.

9. Bring the DBs back up by straightening your elbows; repeat.

exercise 9

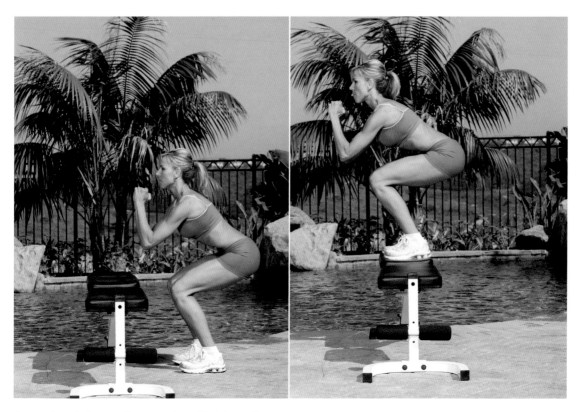

Power bench jumps (legs and cardio interval)

1 Standing in front of the bench, squat down and jump onto the bench with both feet.

2 Jump off the bench, landing in a squat as softly as you can.

3 Repeat the jumps while maintaining a strong upper body.

4 Be very careful not to catch your toes on the sides of the bench.

Repeat exercises 7–9, following your stage 3 calendar guidelines of sets and repetitions

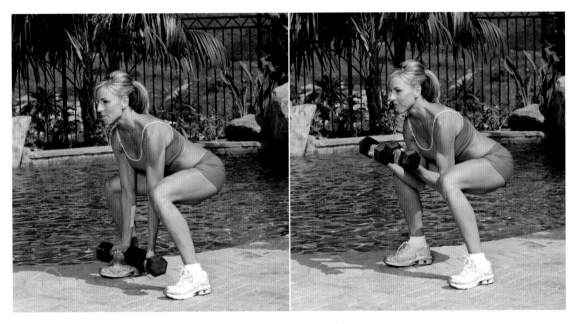

Biceps curl from a squat position (biceps, leg strength, and balance)

1 Hold the DBs in your hands and squat down, keeping a straight back, until your thighs are almost parallel to the floor.

2 Place your elbows on the insides of your knees and extend your arms and DBs toward the floor.

3 With your palms facing up, perform the biceps curl by bringing the DBs to your shoulders and squeezing your biceps.

4 Lower the DBs and repeat the curls, staying in the squatting position.

5 Keep your abs tight and your weight in the heels of your feet to avoid knee injury. Your knees should not come out over your toes; keep your glutes down and back.

exercise 11

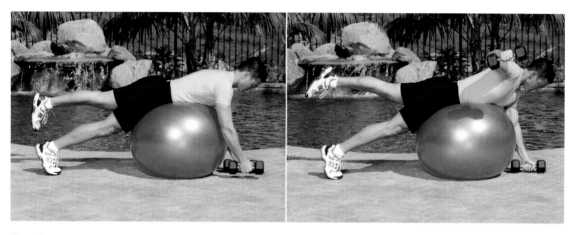

Single arm rear deltoid raise bent over stability ball with single leg lift (shoulders, back, and core)

1. Get on your knees with the DBs in your hands and bring the ball into contact with your torso; maintain contact throughout the exercise.

2. Bring yourself into a prone position by rolling forward so you are on top of the ball.

3. Maintain a neutral spine and keep your head and shoulders up (don't drop your head).

4. If your feet slide, secure them up against a wall or piece of furniture.

5. With the DBs in your hands, squeeze your shoulder blades together.

6. While balancing on the ball, draw your right elbow out to your side and lift your left leg up.

7. Make sure your shoulder and elbow are in line with each other so you activate the rear deltoid.

8. Lower the DB and your leg back down together; repeat.

9. Repeat the exercise with the left arm and right leg.

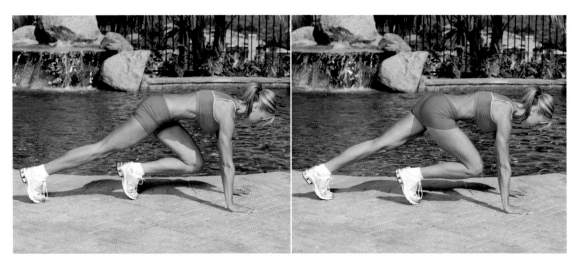

Running man with hands on the floor for 2 minutes

1 Keep your hands on the floor and your body in a push-up position.

2 Bring your knees into your chest, alternating your legs as if you're running.

3 Keep it up for 2 minutes.

4 If this is too difficult or hard on your wrists, you can put your hands on a bench or on a wall.

Repeat exercises 10–12, following your stage 3 calendar guidelines of sets and repetitions

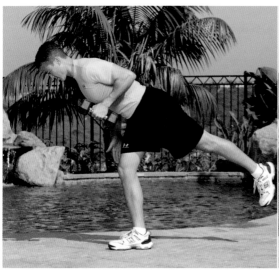 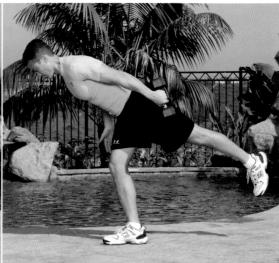

Single leg scale balance with triceps kickback (legs, triceps, and core)

1 Balance on your right leg with a DB in your left hand.

2 Bring yourself into a scale position, trying to bring your torso and left leg parallel to the floor. You may rest your left hand on the bench if you need to maintain your balance.

3 Keep your body long from your head to your toe.

4 Holding that position, take the DB in your left hand and bring your elbow in line with your spine; hold that position.

5 Kick back the right DB and engage your triceps; repeat.

6 Repeat the exercise balancing on your left leg with the right triceps working.

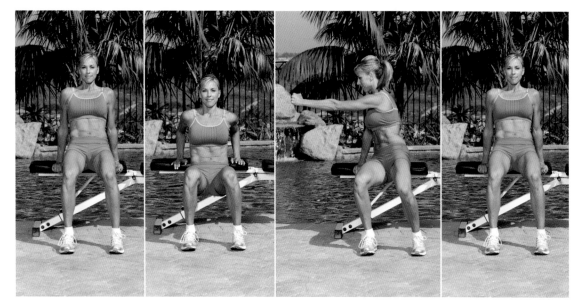

Triceps bench dip into single arm cross punch and torso rotation (triceps, abdominals, and core)

1 Sitting on the floor, place your hands by your sides with your fingertips facing forward.

2 Putting your weight into your arms and hands, lift your hips off the floor.

3 Make sure you keep your shoulders down and back.

4 Concentrating on the back of your upper arms, bend your elbows only, and lower yourself toward the floor.

5 Straighten your elbows to lift the hips back up; as your hips come up, take one hand off the bench and punch across your torso as you rotate to the opposite side. Tighten your abs as you rotate and exhale as you punch.

6 Return your hand to the bench dip position and repeat the punch and twist on the other side.

7 Complete 15 cross punches on each side. That is a total of 30 dips.

exercise 15

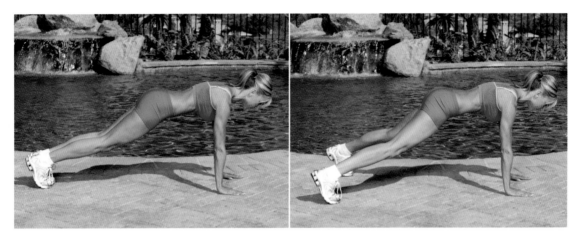

Plank jacks (chest, cardio, and core)

1 Bring yourself into a push-up position; stabilize yourself with your hands under your shoulders and your feet apart.

2 Don't move your hands or torso.

3 Moving only your feet while your upper body remains stable, jump your feet together, then jump them apart, together again, apart, etc.

4 Do a total of 50 reps.

YOU'RE NOW DONE WITH THE STAGE 3, day 2 resistance routine. You did it! Please make sure you stretch and drink plenty of water to stay hydrated. Follow your stage 3 workout calendar for your daily workout plan. Once again, review your goals, track your progress, and keep yourself motivated. Look how far you have come. Keep going! You are on your way to Ultrafitness!

Cardio Exercise Details

Stage 3: Ultrafit Treadmill Blast!

This workout can be performed outside without a machine if you don't have access to a treadmill; you just have to increase your speed if the required incline is unavailable. Using your scale of perceived exertion (scaling effort from 1 to 10), you will need to determine for yourself what slow-, medium-, and fast-paced walking mean to you. When you change speeds and/or inclines, make those transitions as quickly as possible.

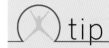

If the workout becomes too difficult for you, bring your effort level down until you are fully recovered and then jump right back into it. Remember to check your heart rate regularly and maintain the appropriate heart rate zone. (I recommend using a heart rate monitor.)

A. WARM-UP: 10 MINUTES			
TIME	FORMAT	PACE	INCLINE
1 Minute	Walk	Medium	Flat
1 Minute	Walk	Fast	Flat
1 Minute	Walk	Medium	3–4%
1 Minute	Walk	Fast	3–4%
1 Minute	Walk	Medium	5–6%
1 Minute	Walk	Fast	5–6%
1 Minute	Walk	Medium	7–8%
1 Minute	Walk	Fast	7–8%
1 Minute	Jog	Medium	Flat
1 Minute	Walk	Medium	Flat

B. WORKING HARD: 10 MINUTES

TIME	FORMAT	PACE	INCLINE
1 Minute	Jog	Medium	Flat
1 Minute	Run	Fast	Flat
1 Minute	Side Shuffle	Medium	Flat (right leg leads)
1 Minute	Side Shuffle	Medium	Flat (left leg leads)
1 Minute	Jog	Medium	Flat
1 Minute	Run	Fast	Flat
1 Minute	Side Shuffle	Medium	Flat (right leg leads)
1 Minute	Side Shuffle	Medium	Flat (left leg leads)
1 Minute	Jog	Medium	Flat
1 Minute	Run	Fast	Flat

20-MINUTE MARK! If your workout ends here, cool down for 1 minute by walking slowly on a flat grade. You're done—now STRETCH!

C. WORKING HARDER: 10 MINUTES

TIME	FORMAT	PACE	INCLINE
1 Minute	Jog	Medium	3–4%
1 Minute	Run	Fast	3–4%
1 Minute	Jog	Medium	5–6%
1 Minute	Run	Fast	5–6%
1 Minute	Jog	Medium	7–8%
1 Minute	Run	Fast	7–8%
1 Minute	Jog	Medium	9–10%
1 Minute	Run	Fast	9–10%
1 Minute	Jog	Medium	Flat
1 Minute	Run	Fast	Flat

30-MINUTE MARK! If your workout ends here, cool down for 1 minute by walking slowly on a flat grade. You're done—now STRETCH!

Stage 3: Ultrafit Stair Challenge

This workout requires a long set of stairs (preferably outside) that are safe to run on. I recommend visiting a local school stadium to see what's available. You can also use a step mill if one is available at your gym.

A. WARM-UP: 5 MINUTES

Run up every step and jog down.

Run up every other step and jog down.

Run up every 3 steps and jog down.

Run up every step and jog down.

Run up every other step and jog down.

Run up every 3 steps and jog down.

Stationary squats for 60 seconds.

Stationary alternating forward lunges for 60 seconds.

B. WORKING HARD: 5 MINUTES

Side run (with right leg leading) up every other step and jog down.

Run up every step and jog down.

Side run (with left leg leading) up every other step and jog down.

Run up every step and jog down.

Bunny hop up (using both legs) every step and jog down.

Run up every step and jog down.

Side run (with right leg leading) up every other step and jog down.

Run up every step and jog down.

Side run (with left leg leading) up every other step and jog down.

Run up every step and jog down.

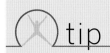

tip

Please note: *If you experience chest pains, lightheadedness or dizziness, nausea, or extreme muscular or joint pain, stop altogether and consult a physician before continuing an exercise program.*

C. WORKING HARDER: 5 MINUTES

Sprint (as fast as you can) up every step and jog down.

Run up every other step and jog down.

On your right leg only, hop up 2 steps, walk up 4 steps, and repeat; jog down.

On your left leg only, hop up 2 steps, walk up 4 steps, and repeat; jog down.

Sprint (as fast as you can) up every step and jog down.

Side squat (with right leg leading) up every other step and jog down.

Side squat (with left leg leading) up every other step and jog down.

Side walk (with left leg leading) up every other step and jog down.

Sprint (as fast as you can) up every step and jog down.

Run up every other step and jog down.

Repeat segments to increase workout time.

15-MINUTE MARK! If your workout ends here, cool down for 1 minute by walking slowly on a flat grade. You're done—now stretch!

Stage 3: Ultrafit Boot Camp

All you need to complete this workout is a good pair of workout shoes and access to outside terrain (preferably on sand, grass, or a running track). Have fun!

A. WARM-UP: 5 MINUTES

Jog forward for 30 seconds.

Jog backward for 30 seconds.

Side shuffle (right leg leading) for 30 seconds.

Side shuffle (left leg leading) for 30 seconds.

Sprint forward as fast as you can for 30 seconds.

Jog backward for 30 seconds.

Sprint forward as fast as you can for 30 seconds.

Jog backward for 30 seconds.

Stop where you are! Complete as many jumping jacks as you can in 60 seconds.

B. WORKING HARD: 5 MINUTES

Bunny hop forward for 30 seconds.

Jog backward for 30 seconds.

Bunny hop forward for 30 seconds.

Stop! Complete as many squat thrusts as you can in 30 seconds.

Keep going! Running man for 30 seconds.

Get up! Sprint as fast as you can for 30 seconds.

Stop where you are! Do as many jump squats as you can in 30 seconds.

Sprint as fast as you can for 30 seconds.

Stop and drop! Complete as many abdominal jackhammers as you can in 30 seconds.

C. WORKING HARDER: 5 MINUTES

Jog forward for 30 seconds.

Transition into forward walking lunges with front kicks for 30 seconds.

Drop down! Do as many bicycle crunches as you can in 30 seconds.

Get up! Forward walking lunges with a back arabesque squeeze for 30 seconds.

Sprint as fast as you can for 30 seconds.

Stop! Complete as many stationary squats as you can in 30 seconds.

Forward frog jump for 30 seconds.

Backward crab crawl for 30 seconds.

Forward frog jump for 30 seconds.

Backward crab crawl for 30 seconds.

Repeat segments to increase workout time.

ARE YOU DONE? Make sure you cool down for at least 60 seconds and stretch.

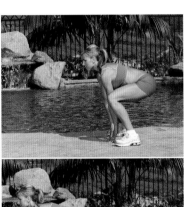

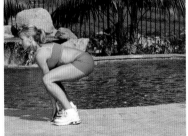

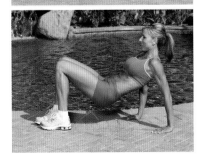

Stage 3: Ultrafit Extreme Jump Rope

This workout requires just a jump rope and you! The best part about this workout is how easily it travels with you, so no excuses!

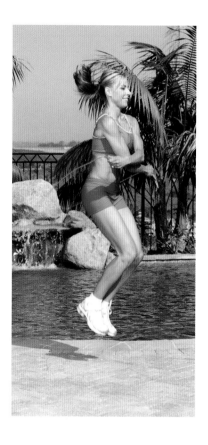

A. WARM-UP: 5 MINUTES

Speed jump rope for 2 minutes.

Slow jump rope for 60 seconds.

Speed jump rope for 2 minutes.

B. WORKING HARD: 5 MINUTES

Alternating double hopping on each foot, jump rope for 60 seconds.

Jump feet in and out with every rope revolution for 60 seconds.

With high knees, jump rope for 60 seconds.

With your left leg only, jump rope for 60 seconds.

With your right leg only, jump rope for 60 seconds.

C. WORKING HARDER: 5 MINUTES

Jump rope with rope cross in front for 60 seconds.

Speed jump rope for 60 seconds.

Jump rope with rope cross in front for 60 seconds.

Speed jump rope for 60 seconds.

Alternating double hopping on each foot, jump rope for 60 seconds.

Repeat segments to increase workout time.

ARE YOU DONE? Make sure you cool down for at least 60 seconds and stretch.

Stage 3: Ultrafit Bike Workout

You will need an outdoor bike, a stationary bike, or a Spin Cycle to complete this workout. You'll need to use your scale of perceived exertion (scaling effort from 1 to 10) combined with adjusting the bike tension on a scale of 1 to 10 throughout the workout.

A. WARM-UP: 10 MINUTES			
TIME	**FORMAT**	**PACE**	**TENSION**
1 Minute	Seated Cycle	Medium	2%
1 Minute	Seated Cycle	Fast	2%
2 Minutes	Climbing Cycle	Medium	2%
1 Minute	Seated Cycle	Medium	4%
1 Minute	Seated Cycle	Fast	4%
2 Minutes	Climbing Cycle	Medium	4%
1 Minute	Seated Cycle	Medium	6%
1 Minute	Seated Cycle	Fast	6%

B. WORKING HARD: 10 MINUTES			
TIME	**FORMAT**	**PACE**	**TENSION**
3 Minutes	Climbing Cycle	Medium	6%
1 Minute	Climbing Cycle	Fast	6%
3 Minutes	Climbing Cycle	Medium	8%
1 Minute	Climbing Cycle	Fast	8%
2 Minutes	Seated Cycle	Fast	10%

20-MINUTE MARK! If your workout ends here, cool down for 1 minute by pedaling slowly with no tension. You're done—now STRETCH!

C. WORKING HARDER: 10 MINUTES

TIME	FORMAT	PACE	TENSION
1 Minute	Seated Cycle	Medium	6%
1 Minute	Seated Cycle	Fast	10%
1 Minute	Seated Cycle	Medium	6%
1 Minute	Seated Cycle	Fast	10%
1 Minute	Seated Cycle	Fast	6%
1 Minute	Climbing Cycle	Fast	10%
1 Minute	Seated Cycle	Fast	6%
1 Minute	Climbing Cycle	Fast	10%
1 Minute	Climbing Cycle	Fast	6%
1 Minute	Climbing Cycle	Fast	10%

30-MINUTE MARK! If your workout ends here, cool down for 1 minute by pedaling slowly with no tension. You're done—now STRETCH!

Stage 3: Ultrafit Sprint Intervals

Just as with the Boot Camp Workout, all you need to complete this workout is a good pair of workout shoes and access to outside terrain (preferably on sand, grass, or a running track). Have fun!

A. WARM-UP: 5 MINUTES

Moderate run for 60 seconds.
Fast run (NOT a sprint) for 60 seconds.
Moderate run for 60 seconds.
Fast run (NOT a sprint) for 60 seconds.
Moderate run for 60 seconds.

B. WORKING HARD: 5 MINUTES

Moderate 20 seconds / fast 20 seconds / sprint 20 seconds speed buildup for a total of 60 seconds.

Slow jog for 30 seconds.

Moderate 20 / fast 20 / sprint 20 speed buildup for a total of 60 seconds.

Slow jog for 30 seconds.

Moderate 20 / fast 20 / sprint 20 speed buildup for a total of 60 seconds.

High knees run for 30 seconds.

Heel kicks run for 30 seconds.

C. WORKING HARDER: 5 MINUTES

Suicide runs: Select three points in a straight line progressively farther away. Sprint to the first, run back to the start; sprint to the second, run back to the start; sprint to the third, and run back to the start.

Repeat 3 times.

Repeat segments to increase workout time.

Time to cool down and stretch!

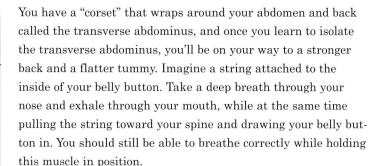

You have a "corset" that wraps around your abdomen and back called the transverse abdominus, and once you learn to isolate the transverse abdominus, you'll be on your way to a stronger back and a flatter tummy. Imagine a string attached to the inside of your belly button. Take a deep breath through your nose and exhale through your mouth, while at the same time pulling the string toward your spine and drawing your belly button in. You should still be able to breathe correctly while holding this muscle in position.

Equipment Needed

- Hand weights
- Stability ball

Exercise Format

- There are 4 super-sets of exercises (exercises to be performed back to back), each to be completed 3 times before moving on to the next super-set.

tip

It's extremely important that you breathe correctly and, at the same time, properly draw in your abdominal muscles prior to engaging in any of these exercises.

suggestions and definitions

This abdominal workout has been designed to target your entire "core" area. When I mention an "isometric" move (e.g., "V-sit isometric hold"), it actually refers to no movement at all. Isometric training requires you to sustain a muscle contraction over a given period of time, and there are no repetitions required.

The end result of isometric training is that the muscle begins to recruit and activate more motor units to help maintain this contraction, and the motor units are then forced to contract continuously, time after time, thus maturing the entire muscle very quickly.

exercise 1

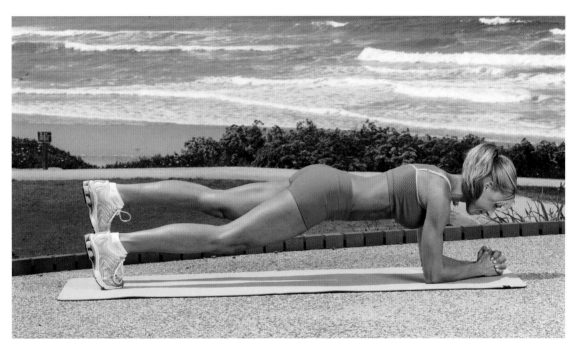

Plank hold from forearms with single leg up for 30 seconds

1 Get down on the floor on your hands and knees.

2 Bring yourself down so that you are resting on your forearms.

3 Make sure your shoulders are directly over your elbows and clasp your hands together.

4 Tighten up those abs and keep your spine long.

5 Extend both your legs so that your knees are off the ground and your toes are supporting you.

6 Your body should be straight from the tip of your head all the way through to your feet.

7 Make sure you don't drop into your shoulders or arch your back; maintain shoulder girdle stability.

8 Take your left leg off the ground and hold for 30 seconds.

9 Return your left leg to the starting position and repeat with your right leg in the air for the next 30 seconds with no breaks in between.

10 Challenge: If this gets easy, you can try the same move with your toes on a stability ball and your hands on the floor.

exercise 2

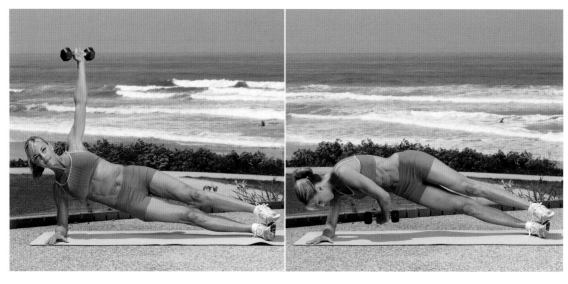

Side plank oblique dumbbell rotation; 30 reps

1 Place one DB of medium size on the ground and bring yourself into the forearm plank hold as described earlier.

2 Bring your forearms together so they are touching, parallel to each other, and each hand is touching the opposite elbow.

3 Roll yourself onto your right elbow with your shoulder directly over the elbow; you'll now be looking at the wall instead of the floor.

4 Make sure your hips are stacked on top of each other and your feet are stacked or staggered with the left foot in front of the right. Stacked is more difficult.

5 Grab the DB with your left hand and extend your left arm up to the ceiling, opening your chest. This is your starting point.

6 Engage your abs as you slowly bring the DB in your left hand down androtate your torso as you go.

7 Stop the rotation when you feel your obliques engage. Try not to slouch into your shoulders, and hold your abs in during the entire exercise.

8 Repeat the side plank DB rotation for 15 reps on the right side and then 15 on the left.

Repeat exercises 1 and 2 for 3 sets

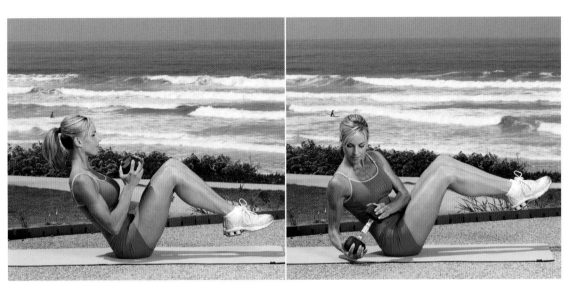

V-sit dumbbell rotation; 30 reps

1 Sit on the floor holding one DB by your chest and bring your knees up with your feet off the floor.

2 Make sure your chest is lifted, your shoulders are back, and those abs are really tight.

3 Keep your back as straight as possible.

4 Balancing in the "V" position, rotate to the right with the DB, come back to center, and then rotate to the left. Complete 15 reps on each side.

exercise 4

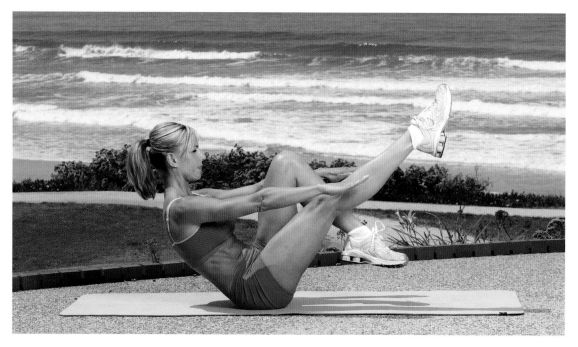

V-sit with alternating leg extension; 30 reps

1 Sit on the floor, bringing your knees to your chest with your feet off the floor.

2 Make sure your chest is lifted, your shoulders are back, and those abs are really tight.

3 Keeping your back as straight as possible, extend your left leg out and up so your body takes the shape of a "V."

4 Reach your arms straight in front of you and hold.

5 Bring your left leg in, straighten your right leg, and hold.

6 Alternate the left leg and then the right leg for 15 reps on each side.

Repeat exercises 3 and 4 for 3 sets

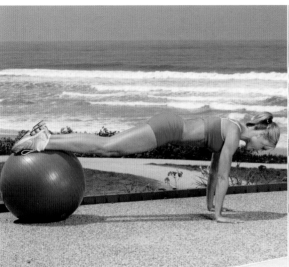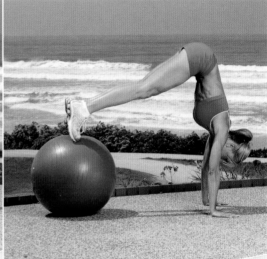

Pike roll on stability ball; 15 reps

1 Get on your knees with the ball in front of you.

2 Roll yourself over the ball and then begin to walk your hands out and away.

3 Walk yourself out into a push-up position with a neutral spine, tight abs, and shoulder girdle stability.

4 Challenge: The farther out you walk your hands, the harder the exercise will be.

5 Find a position you can maintain and hold it with your hands shoulder width apart.

6 Keeping your weight in your hands, push your toes into the stability ball, engage your core, and drive your hips straight up toward the ceiling as high as you can get them with your toes straight down on the ball.

7 You must keep your legs straight to make this a true pike.

8 Roll the stability ball toward your shoulders.

9 Lower yourself back down slowly into the push-up position and repeat.

exercise 6

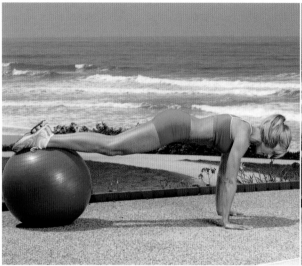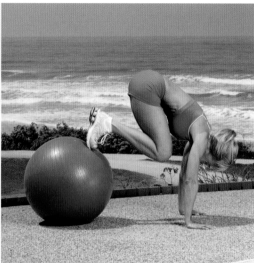

Reverse crunch roll with stability ball; 25 reps

1 Get on your knees with the ball in front of you.

2 Roll yourself over the ball and then begin to walk your hands out and away.

3 Walk yourself out into a push-up position with a neutral spine, tight abs, and shoulder girdle stability.

4 Challenge: The farther out you walk your hands, the harder the exercise will be.

5 Find a position you can maintain and hold it with your hands shoulder width apart.

6 Keeping your weight in your hands, push your shins into the stability ball and begin to bend your knees and draw them into your chest.

7 Try to keep your toes parallel to the floor as your draw in, ending with your toes straight down on the stability ball.

8 Push the stability ball back out into the push-up position with your legs straight; repeat.

Repeat exercises 5 and 6 for 3 sets

Great job! Now remember to stretch. Lying on the ball with your arms stretched out to your sides and your feet planted on the floor is a great way to stretch out your abdominal area.

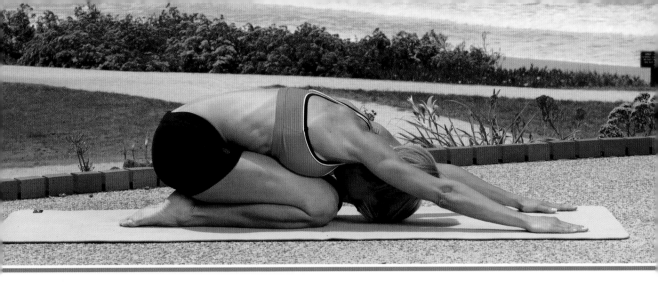

ultrafit stretch series

Flexibility training is an important part of your workout routine. It should not be ignored. Being flexible helps prevent injuries, improves joint integrity, releases stress, and so much more. The following exercises are my own version of yoga and stretching. I am not a yoga instructor, by any means, but this is the series of stretches that I like to do. I feel they are very effective if they are done consistently. I love Glenda Twining's book, *Yoga Turns Back the Clock*. There are very easy but practical poses and stretches in this great book. I recommend it.

There are all kinds of yoga courses designed specifically for beginners as well as for advanced students, and prenatal classes are offered in some gyms as well. There are also many yoga and stretching videos on the market. In my *10-Minute Solution, Target Toning* video, I have a great 10-minute power stretch at the end. You will need a mat for this stretch series.

I like to stretch after my cardio workout so my body is completely warmed up. If your calendar calls for weights, cardio, and stretching, do your weights first, cardio second, and stretch last. Hold each stretch for 1 minute. If you do that, the stretch series should take approximately 20 minutes. You can repeat desired stretches to make it longer or if you need extra flexibility in one particular area.

Stretching is most effective when used as part of your warm-up. In fact, exercising without properly stretching in advance is a common cause of injury.

exercise 1

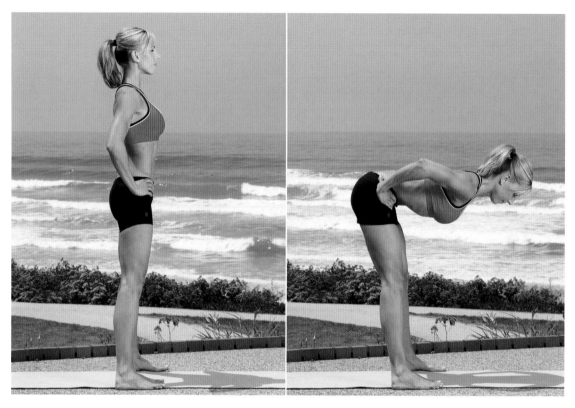

Wide-angle forward bend for 60 seconds

1. Start by standing with your legs wider than shoulder width apart and your toes slightly turned in.

2. Place your thumbs on the back of your hips with your elbows facing behind you.

3. Keeping your legs straight and engaging your abs, inhale and exhale while bending over from the hips as far as you can go while keeping your back straight and your spine and neck in a neutral position.

4. You should feel a stretch in your hamstrings, glutes, and lower back.

5. Hold this position for 60 seconds.

6. Challenge: If you want to take this stretch deeper, release your hands from your hips, reach down, and grab your big toe on each foot. Hold here for 60 seconds.

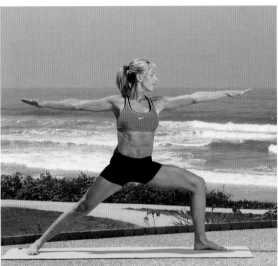 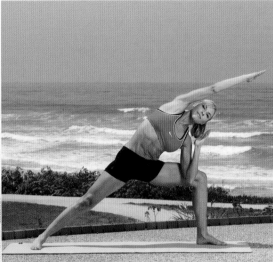

Extended side lunge for 60 seconds

1. Start by bending your left knee, toes facing your knee, so it is directly above your ankle, forming a 90-degree angle, and lower yourself into a lunge position. Your right toes should be facing outward, away from your body. Keep your hips aligned. Your arms should be stretched out parallel to the floor and in the same direction as your legs.

2. Inhale and bend from the right side of your torso, bringing your left elbow to the inside of your left knee. Press against the left knee with your left elbow and open your chest by extending your right arm up and over your head and pressing your right shoulder back.

3. You should feel this throughout your entire body but specifically in your legs, back, inner and outer thighs, glutes, shoulders, and neck.

4. Hold this position and breathe slowly in and out for 60 seconds.

exercise 3

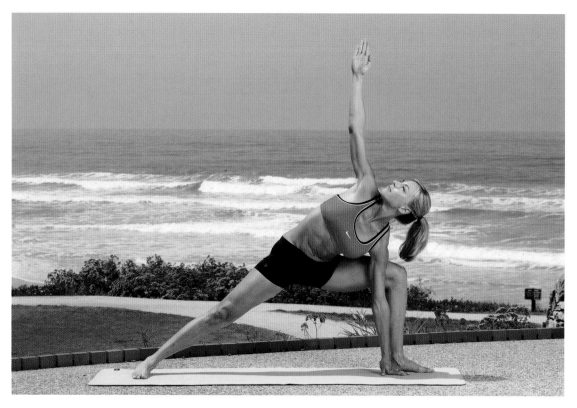

Extended side-angle pose for 60 seconds

1 From the extended side lunge position, inhale, then exhale while dropping your left hand to the ground and sliding your right leg even further into the stretch.

2 Make sure your left knee still does not extend out over your toes. At the same time, extend your right arm, reaching for the ceiling, and look up toward your right arm.

3 This is a deeper stretch than the extended side lunge, so if you are comfortable in that stretch you may stay there for 2 minutes instead of taking it further into this stretch. You will gradually get more flexible, so be patient.

Repeat stretches 1–3, changing sides on stretches 2 and 3, for a total of 6 minutes

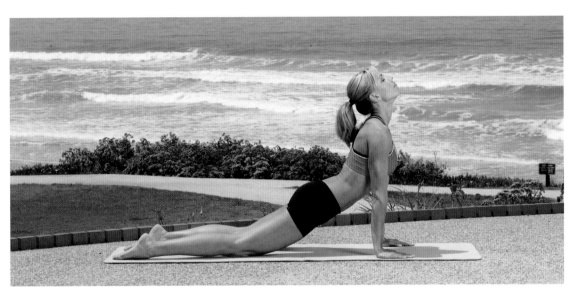

Upward-facing dog for 60 seconds

1 Inhale, bring your arms over your head, exhale, and bring your hands and palms down to the floor on the outside of your feet, bending your knees if necessary.

2 Tuck your chin and lock your elbows to support your body and jump both feet back or step them back separately. Exhaling, straighten your legs and elbows while tightening your abdominal muscles.

3 Lower yourself to the floor, keeping your torso straight, then come into an arched position with your chest on the floor and your elbows lifted.

4 Inhaling, slide your body forward and up. Exhaling, drop your hips to the floor, press your arms straight, stretch up through your head, and arch your back. Keep your legs together and press the tops of your feet into the floor. Imagine that you are trying to push your hips through your elbows to increase the arch in your back.

5 Arch your spine and gaze directly in front of you or gently drop your head back.

6 Hold this pose for 60 seconds.

7 If you want more of a challenge, lift your hips off the floor for a deeper stretch.

8 This stretch will open your chest, stretch your back, and strengthen your arms and shoulders.

exercises
5&6

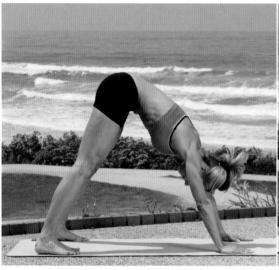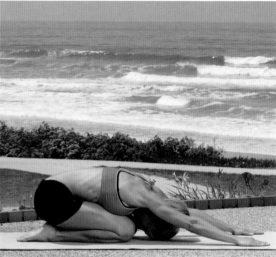

Downward-facing dog

Child's pose, arms extended

1 Starting from the upward-facing dog position, curl your toes under and lift your hips. Stretch back into downward-facing dog, transferring your weight back toward your heels.

2 Your glutes will be up in the air like an inverted V. Press your heels down and lift your glutes up so you feel a deep stretch in your glutes, hamstrings, back, neck, and upper body.

3 Hold the pose for 60 seconds.

1 Kneel on the floor and bring your glutes toward your heels.

2 Reach and stretch your arms out in front of your body and place them on the floor in front of you.

3 Stretch your chin forward and gently lower your forehead to the floor, rounding your spine and shoulders.

4 Relax your neck muscles and relax into the pose. Hold the pose for 60 seconds.

Repeat stretches 4 through 6 twice, for a total of 6 minutes

exercise 7

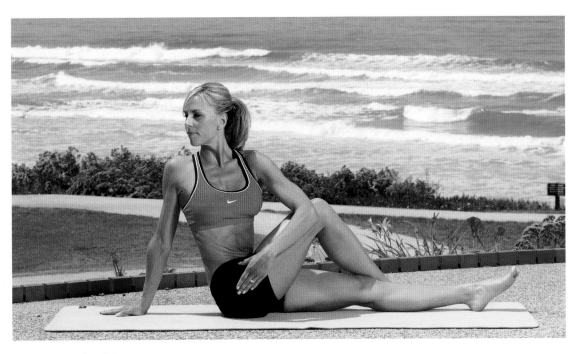

Seated spinal twist

1. Sit tall, with your spine as straight as you can and both legs extended forward.

2. Raise your right knee and place your right foot on the floor; allow your left leg to remain flat.

3. Place your right hand flat on the floor behind you, not too far from your body; try not to lean, but twist instead.

4. Raise your left arm and bring it over the right side of your right knee; bend your elbow, pressing against your knee, and place your hand on your thigh.

5. Hold this position and slowly inhale and exhale while twisting a bit deeper into the stretch.

6. Hold for 60 seconds and then switch sides.

exercise 8

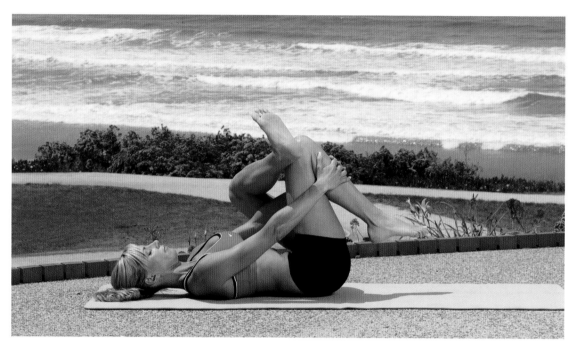

Lying down hip stretch

1 Lie flat on your back with the sole of your right foot flat on the floor.

2 Place your left ankle on top of your right knee and flex your left foot.

3 Wrap your hands around your right knee and interlace your fingers.

4 Challenge: The closer you bring your knee to your chest, the greater the stretch in your hips will be.

5 Hold the stretch for 60 seconds while slowly inhaling and exhaling. Switch sides.

Repeat stretches 7 and 8 twice, for a total of 4 minutes

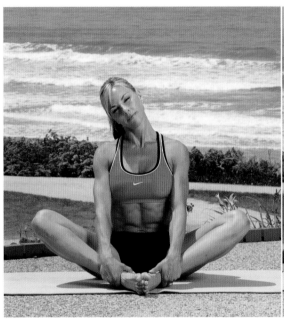 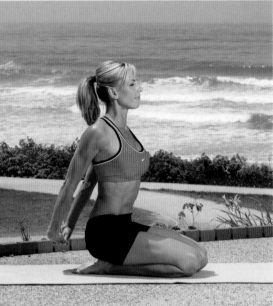

Butterfly inner thigh stretch and neck release   **Kneeling arms and shoulder stretch**

1 Sit with your back tall and straight; bring the bottoms of your feet together and your knees out wide.

2 Pull your heels in as close as you can to your body while holding on to your ankles; gently press down on your knees with your elbows to feel a deep stretch in your inner thighs.

3 Drop your head sideways to the right until you feel a comfortable stretch in your neck on the left side. Hold this stretch for 60 seconds with your head to the right, and then switch sides with your head to the left for 60 seconds.

1 Kneel on the floor with your back tall and straight, and then gently sit your glutes down on your heels. Interlace your fingers behind your back.

2 With you shoulders pushed back and your arms straight, lift your arms as high as you can, feeling a good stretch in your arms and shoulders. Hold this pose for 60 seconds.

3 **NOTE:** If it hurts your knees to sit back on your heels, do the stretch from a kneeling position.

Repeat stretches 9 and 10 twice, for a total of 4 minutes

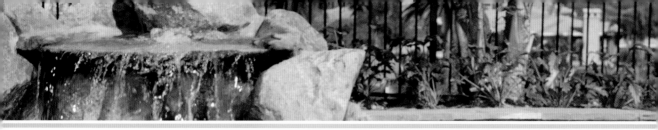

CHAPTER 8
ultrafit nutrition

MY GUIDELINES FOR SUCCESS

I am a licensed sports nutritionist and a certified lifestyle and weight management consultant. It has always been my goal to educate my clients on how to create positive eating habits that will fit in with their typically busy schedules. It's important that you understand how and why this program works; I want you to serve as an example of change that will influence and motivate family and friends to do the same.

My program is not just a diet but also a complete change of lifestyle and behavior. Like everything in life, moderation is the key. I think there is a difference in eating to be healthy, eating to lose weight, and eating to be healthy and lean. There are diets out there that tell you to eat whatever you want but only in small amounts. There are diets that tell you it is okay to eat all the protein and fat you want. There are also liquid diets and fasting diets. My theory is this: No matter which diet you do, the bottom line is calories in versus calories out. You need to eat less and move more—plain and simple. That is why I use lower calories in the beginning to teach portion control and to help you see results right away. I ask you to be strict when it comes to sugar, saturated fat, and processed foods for a period of time until you increase your metabolism and your body becomes a natural fat-burning machine.

Saturated fat is bad for your heart and for your weight. It will clog your arteries and cause unwanted weight gain. Fat is very important to have in your diet, but it has to be the right kind

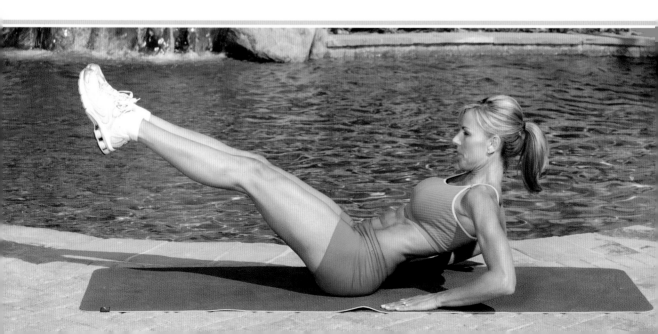

of fat. Unsaturated, polyunsaturated, and monounsaturated fats are the kinds to look for. I ask my clients to keep their saturated fat amount to less than 10 percent of their total calories. I promote eating good fats, such as almonds, walnuts, small amounts of olive oil, some dairy fat, fish, and lean proteins. I also have my clients take Ultrafit-Omega Oil, an oil combination of 8 essential fatty acids, every day for hormone regulation, blood sugar regulation, immune system strength, joint therapy, and moisture for skin, hair, and nails. This ensures they are getting enough good fat in their diets without getting the saturated fat from their foods. I also have them take food "pacs," which are tablets that contain water-soluble nutrients that have been extracted from real food.

The foods you eat must provide good calories for your body to increase muscle, lose fat, and get lean. It is important to have a good blend of complex carbohydrates, lean proteins, fibrous vegetables, fruits, and good fats throughout the day. Processed foods and "white foods" that contain white flour or white sugar have the same effect on blood sugar as regular sugar does. They cause a rapid rise in blood sugar, thus causing your body to make extra insulin to bring the blood back to a state of homeostasis. This causes your body to feel tired, to get hungry faster, and, if you have too much sugar, to store it as fat. The more unprocessed the food, the better it is for your body's health and leanness.

I believe sugar is one of the worst things that you can put into your body.

There is no right diet answer for everyone. What I've outlined in this book is what works for me and for 95 percent of my clients. The reason my programs have helped so many people accomplish their health and fitness goals is because Ultrafit is easy, balanced, and simple to follow.

The principles behind my program are to increase your metabolism by drinking more water, eating small meals every 3 to 4 hours, adding weight resistance to your workouts to help increase lean muscle mass, and not going overboard with the cardio (spending hours sweating it out without a real plan will lead to boredom and, very often, failure).

ESSENTIAL ELEMENTS FOR SUCCESS

There are four elements that, if followed, will ensure that my Ultrafit program works for you:

1. Attitude and adherence
2. Planning ahead
3. Staying hydrated
4. Cutting out the junk

Attitude and Adherence

First, get excited! To make a lifestyle change, you have to look forward to what you are doing, as well as what you have the ability to accomplish. These programs have been specifically designed to avoid the usual feelings of exhaustion and frustration that a radical new program can bring on. In addition to a new progressive exercise routine, I'm suggesting a healthy eating plan that you carry into your everyday life once you have accomplished the initial metabolic transformations your body needs to function more effectively.

Second, don't stray! If you want to achieve maximum results in a relatively short period of time, you must follow the programs as closely as possible. I'm asking you to make a strong com-

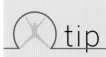

mitment both to my Ultrafit program and to yourself. It takes the body 4 to 6 weeks to make a change in its fat-burning engine (the metabolism), so the stricter you are in the beginning, the more you will accomplish in the long run. Once your metabolism has been raised, the once-in-a-while "special-occasion" diet splurge will not make as much of a difference. (As long as you don't overdo it!)

Planning Ahead

The objectives of my Ultrafit program are to keep your body in a comfortable hormonal balance all day long. This requires you to have greater control over hormonal fluctuations and insulin levels, and you can easily accomplish this by eating the right foods at the right times throughout the day. You may think that the best way to lose weight is to starve yourself and limit your food intake, but just the opposite is true.

The solution to maximizing your hormonal response, jump-starting your metabolism, and controlling your weight is in proper meal timing. While following the Ultrafit exercise program, you must also establish a healthy and consistent dietary routine. This means eating every 3 to 4 hours (two snacks and three meals), controlling portion sizes, and cutting out the junk. Now, this is obviously easier said than done, especially with the typical busy schedules that many of us keep. Therefore, it is absolutely essential that you plan ahead. Get yourself to the grocery store before your cupboards go bare and you resort to snacking or fast food. Prepare meals ahead of time and bring them with you. Keep healthy snacks at the office, in your car, wherever! Do what you have to do to make sure you're never in a situation that leaves you with little or no options. Keep an accurate food diary so that you are aware of your caloric intake. If you aren't able to stick to my caloric recommendations because you didn't take the time to think about your needs during the day, the only result you'll have is disappointment when you come to the end of your program.

Staying Hydrated

Depending on your program, your ultimate goal is to take in between 60 and 128 ounces of water each day. I suggest that for a short period of time you eliminate all juices, regular/diet sodas, and sugared/flavored drinks from your diet, and if you choose to consume them, you do so in strict moderation. Beverages with caffeine should be limited as well, because they only serve to dehydrate you due to their diuretic effects. It's important (especially when exercising) that you don't wait until you're thirsty to drink water. Once you feel thirsty, you're already dehydrated, and when we're dehydrated, our brains often incorrectly signal that we're hungry. Not only will drinking sufficient amounts of water keep you looking and feeling better, but it will also keep the hunger pangs at bay and prevent you from unnecessary, "mindless" snacking.

Cutting Out the Junk

By eating well-balanced meals on a regular schedule, you're balancing your blood-sugar levels and preventing any sudden spikes or drops in insulin levels. Any additional dietary sugar can knock that balance completely out of whack. So the key is to keep your sugar intake low. A simple way to identify hidden sugars in processed foods is to look for words ending in "ose" (e.g., glucose, lactose, sucrose), and if any of these words appear in the first three ingredients listed, then the item is likely to be high in sugar and should be avoided.

As for dietary fat, I want to reiterate what I said earlier about fat. I want you to understand that although there are "good" fats out there that your body needs, they still need to be consumed in strict moderation during the first phases of your new lifestyle change. You'll be safe if you stick with the monounsaturated fats such as canola oil and olive oil, and polyunsaturated fats such as corn oil, peanut oil, and sesame oil. Fats to avoid are those classified as hydrogenated or saturated, as well as any trans-fatty acids (whenever possible). I personally take an oil combination of essential fatty acids every day along with all-natural food-based nutrients. This assures me that I am getting my fat-soluble and water-soluble nutrients every day. I strongly recommend this to all my clients as well. I suggest you do research to determine which supplements are right for you.

As you begin to see results, build on your motivation, which will increase your willpower.

DETERMINING YOUR NUTRITIONAL NEEDS

Remember in chapter 3 when you determined your body-fat composition? Now, to determine your recommended caloric intake, you must determine your resting metabolic rate (RMR):

> Resting Metabolic Rate (RMR) =
> 413 + (Lean Body Mass in lbs. x 0.4536)

RMR is typically 70 to 80 percent of the average person's total energy expenditure. Therefore, a good place to start is with RMR or RMR plus 10 percent. For example, if your RMR is 1500, you should be consuming around 1500 calories a day; if you are a more active person (see the activity level descriptions on the next page), then you could add 10 percent to your total calorie amount. That would be an additional 150 calories, making your total calories 1650.

I use RMR in my practice all the time to determine the specific caloric intake for my clients. I have a metabolic testing machine that I feel is very accurate. But because you might not have access to this type of machine, the previous formula is a good way to estimate your total calories. However, nothing is more important than listening to your body's needs and using common sense to determine your appropriate caloric intake level, especially as workouts grow in both intensity and duration. You must be willing to be flexible, and it's extremely important that you take the time to recalculate your body fat at set points in your program (e.g., 6 weeks, 12 weeks, and 18 weeks). This will ensure that you are on the correct path to Ultrafitness.

Activity Level Descriptions

Use the following descriptions to determine your activity level. Remember, if you are in the moderate to extremely heavy activity levels, you should definitely add 10 percent to your total caloric intake.

1. **Sedentary activity:** This is mainly sitting at a desk all day. You rarely experience any physical activity throughout the day.

2. **Light activity:** This includes continuous exercise, such as walking approximately three times per week for approximately 20 minutes each session. If you are not involved in regular activity, you may be on your feet all day through work (e.g., working as a waitress). Daily activities may include regular walking.

3. **Moderate activity:** This involves continuous exercise three or more times per week for more than 20-minute sessions. Walking at a brisk pace, dancing, working in the yard, jogging, and swimming are all examples.

4. **Heavy activity:** This is continuous exercise three to five times per week for approximately 60-minute sessions. It involves a lot of physical activity for an extended period and may include heavy-labor jobs, such as construction.

5. **Extremely heavy activity:** This is continuous exercise five or more times per week for sessions lasting 60 minutes or more. It involves a lot of physical activity for an extended period and may include heavy-labor jobs, such as construction.

MY ULTRAFIT NUTRITION SYSTEMS' SAMPLE MENUS

This chapter is dedicated to giving you an example of how I eat and how my clients eat to lose weight and decrease body fat. I've put together two sample daily meal plans, one for men and one for women, with calorie amounts set to help you achieve Ultrafitness. Each day is between 1300 and 1400 calories for women and 2100 for men. You should adjust the calories according to the formula we discussed earlier in the chapter. These are only suggestions, so please feel free to make exchanges for foods you don't like or foods you don't have access to.

In addition, you can check out my Web site, www.ultranutrition.com, for recipes that adhere to the Ultrafit requirements. If you want more healthy Ultrafit recipes, my cookbook, Ultrafit Cooking, can be found on the Web site as well.

I have put a sample food log after the menu for you to copy and use for your entire program. I find logging what you eat a great way to maintain a healthy diet. If you have to write it down, you'll be more selective of what you eat.

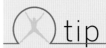

Everyday, be sure to eat or drink:

- *Essential fatty acids*
- *A wide range of nutrients*
- *Plenty of water*

the ultrafit list of dos and don'ts

Ultrafit Dos

- DO drink more water. The range, depending upon an individual's age and activity level, is ideally between 60 and 128 ounces of water per day.
- DO consider taking essential fatty acids (EFA) along with water-soluble nutrients or a multivitamin that together complete your fat-soluble and water-soluble nutrient needs.
- DO eat every three hours, having five or six small meals a day. Try to keep all meals the same amount of calories. No skipping or snacking!
- DO follow both a cardio program and a weights program within one of the Ultrafit calendars as closely as possible.
- DO feel free to combine programs from different levels (e.g., intermediate weights and advanced cardio).
- DO take the time to treat your body to a good stretch and at least one day off a week. This means listening to your body.
- DO eat fruit. If you are trying to lose weight, limit the amount of fruit you eat to one or two pieces per day. Try to choose fruits high in fiber and antioxidants and low in sugar, and always add in a protein and a good fat source to slow the digestion process.
- DO eat two complex carbohydrates per day (preferably at breakfast or lunch), combining them with a protein and a fat source. For example, oatmeal, protein powder, and five almonds would be a great breakfast.
- DO feel comfortable going out to eat. Choose lean protein sources such as chicken, fish, or turkey, or small amounts of lean red meat, and request that it be grilled, baked, poached, or steamed, with sauce on the side; have a large salad with nonfat or low-fat dressing on the side (or just balsamic vinegar); limit alcohol to one drink; make sure you eat cheese, butter, or any type of white sauce in moderation; choose brown rice or plain baked potato instead of bread; and stick to sampling other people's desserts rather than ordering your own.
- DO try to plan what you're going to eat each day, and what you need to bring with you, the night before; avoid making poor meal choices or going on food binges because of lack of planning.
- DO take bottled water, healthy snacks, and essential nutrients on trips away from home (including when you're traveling to and from home in your car).

Ultrafit Don'ts

- DON'T try to make up for skipped workouts or overeating by going crazy with the cardio; your body doesn't work that way, and you won't see any real improvements by needlessly exhausting yourself.
- DON'T ignore physical pains or problems, and be sure to schedule an appointment with your physician before embarking on a new fitness and nutrition program.
- DON'T skip the weight-training days in any of the Ultrafit programs; you must develop lean muscle mass to see positive changes in your body.
- DON'T consume simple sugars, sweets, white flour, and processed foods (whenever possible).
- DON'T include processed foods containing hydrogenated oils and fats in your diet.
- DON'T overdo it on salad dressing; stick to 2 to 3 tablespoons of low-fat dressing and use that for your fat source for your meal. If you already have a fat source in the meal, then be sure to use a nonfat dressing, and always have a restaurant bring it on the side so you can see how much is being used.
- DON'T eat two to three hours before going to bed.
- DON'T drink more than one beverage with caffeine a day. I recommend drinking green tea.
- DON'T drink any sodas of any kind.
- DON'T eat more than one protein bar a day; try to keep the sugar content in any protein bar to less than 9 grams, and eat only half a bar at a sitting.
- DON'T eat or drink food with aspartame; try Stevia or Splenda instead.
- DON'T consume more than 30 percent of your total calories in a day in fat. Twenty to 30 grams of fat per day is a good range, and limit your saturated fat to 10 percent of your total daily intake.
- DON'T consume Olestra, the fat substitute that can cause loose stools and abdominal cramping.
- DON'T set unrealistic expectations for yourself. This will only frustrate and de-motivate you. These programs require patience and dedication. You can do it!

WOMEN'S SAMPLE MENU

Breakfast

QTY	MEASURE	DESCRIPTION	PROTEIN (gm)	CARBS (gm)	FAT (gm)	CALORIES
1	oz	Cheddar cheese, reduced fat	8 gm	1 gm	5 gm	80 cal
4	each	Egg whites, scrambled or boiled	14 gm	1.2 gm	0gm	68 cal
2	Tbsp	Mild salsa	.24 gm	1.64 gm	.09 gm	8 cal
1/4	cup	Vegetables, mixed, frozen, boiled	1.3 gm	5.95 gm	.05 gm	27 cal
1	Tbsp	Essential fatty acids oil			12 gm	120 cal
		SUBTOTALS:	23.54 gm	9.79 gm	17.14 gm	303 cal

Morning snack

QTY	MEASURE	DESCRIPTION	PROTEIN (gm)	CARBS (gm)	FAT (gm)	CALORIES
1	oz	Turkey breast	8.5 gm	0.00	.20 gm	38.25 cal
15	each	Almonds	3.19 gm	2.96 gm	7.6 gm	87 cal
1	each	Apple	.30 gm	21.1 gm	0 gm	81 cal
		SUBTOTALS:	11.99 gm	24.06 gm	7.8 gm	206.25 cal

Lunch

QTY	MEASURE	DESCRIPTION	PROTEIN (gm)	CARBS (gm)	FAT (gm)	CALORIES
5	each	Carrot, raw mini	.05 gm	6 gm	.5 gm	30 cal
1	Tbsp	Mayonnaise, fat-free	0 gm	3 gm	0 gm	8 cal
3/4	cup	Tuna in water	45 gm	0 gm	3 gm	210 cal
5	each	Whole wheat crackers, low salt	2.14 gm	15.7 gm	2.14 gm	86 cal
		SUBTOTALS:	47.19 gm	24.7 gm	5.64 gm	334 cal

Afternoon snack

QTY	MEASURE	DESCRIPTION	PROTEIN (gm)	CARBS (gm)	FAT (gm)	CALORIES
5	each	Almonds	1.28 gm	1.18 gm	3.04 gm	34.68 cal
1/2	cup	Nonfat cottage cheese	18 gm	5 gm	0 gm	80 cal
4	oz	Yogurt, low-fat	4.67 gm	22 gm	0 gm	107 cal
		SUBTOTALS:	23.95 gm	28.18 gm	3.04 gm	221.68 cal

Dinner

QTY	MEASURE	DESCRIPTION	PROTEIN (gm)	CARBS (gm)	FAT (gm)	CALORIES
1/2	cup	Refried beans, fat-free	6 gm	18 gm	0 gm	100 cal
1	each	Chicken taco	24 gm	33 gm	7 gm	197 cal
		SUBTOTALS:	30 gm	51 gm	7 gm	297 cal
		ACTUAL TOTALS:	**136.67 gm**	**137.73 gm**	**40.62 gm**	**1361.93 cal**

MEN'S SAMPLE MENU

Breakfast

QTY	MEASURE	DESCRIPTION	PROTEIN (gm)	CARBS (gm)	FAT (gm)	CALORIES
2	oz	Cheddar cheese, shredded, reduced-fat	16 gm	2 gm	10 gm	160 cal
3	each	Egg whites, scrambled or boiled	10.5 gm	.9 gm	0 gm	51 cal
1	each	Egg, whole with yolk	8 gm	1 gm	5 gm	90 cal
2	Tbsp	Mild salsa	.24 gm	1.64 gm	.09 gm	8 cal
1/4	cup	Vegetables, mixed, frozen, boiled	1.3 gm	5.95 gm	.05 gm	27 cal
1 1/2	Tbsp	Essential fatty acids oil			18 gm	180 cal
		SUBTOTALS:	36.04 gm	11.49 gm	33.14 gm	516 cal

Morning snack

QTY	MEASURE	DESCRIPTION	PROTEIN (gm)	CARBS (gm)	FAT (gm)	CALORIES
2	oz	Turkey breast	17 gm	0 gm	.40 gm	76.50 cal
20	each	Almonds	4.25 gm	3.95 gm	10.13 gm	116 cal
1	each	Apple	.30 gm	21.1 gm	0 gm	81 cal
		SUBTOTALS:	21.55 gm	25.05 gm	10.53 gm	273.5 cal

Lunch

QTY	MEASURE	DESCRIPTION	PROTEIN (gm)	CARBS (gm)	FAT (gm)	CALORIES
6	each	Carrot, raw mini	.06 gm	7.2 gm	.6 gm	36 cal
12	each	Whole wheat crackers, low salt	5.14 gm	37.71 gm	5.14 gm	206 cal
1	Tbsp	Mayonnaise, fat-free	0 gm	3 gm	0 gm	8 cal
3/4	cup	Tuna in water	45 gm	0 gm	3 gm	210 cal
		SUBTOTALS:	50.20 gm	47.91 gm	8.74 gm	460 cal

Afternoon snack

QTY	MEASURE	DESCRIPTION	PROTEIN (gm)	CARBS (gm)	FAT (gm)	CALORIES
5	each	Almonds	1.25 gm	1.18 gm	3.04 gm	34.68 cal
2 1/2	cup	Cottage cheese, nonfat	36 gm	10 gm	0 gm	160 cal
6	oz	Yogurt, low-fat	7 gm	33 gm	0 gm	160 cal
		SUBTOTALS:	44.25 gm	44.18 gm	3.04 gm	354.68 cal

Dinner

QTY	MEASURE	DESCRIPTION	PROTEIN (gm)	CARBS (gm)	FAT (gm)	CALORIES
3	oz	Chicken breast, white meat	26.40 gm	0 gm	3 gm	140 cal
1 1/2	cup	Refried beans, fat-free	6 gm	18 gm	0 gm	100 cal
2	each	Chicken tacos	24 gm	33 gm	7 gm	297 cal
		SUBTOTALS:	56.40 gm	51 gm	10 gm	537 cal
		ACTUAL TOTALS:	**208.44 gm**	**179.63 gm**	**65.45 gm**	**2141.18 cal**

Sample Food Log

This is your sample food log. If you can make copies of this and use it for 6 weeks I think it will help. It is also good to write down your moods or situations that occur when you eat. If you are someone who binge eats, be sure to write down what is going on in your life or the mood you are in when you do. That way, you can figure out your triggers and maybe recognize—and stop—a pattern. See chapter 9 for more information.

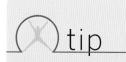

Check out the Ultrafit Web site for all sorts of specially designed recipes to help keep you fit. You'll find dozens at www.ultrafitnutrition.com.

MONDAY:_____	WATER:_____	WORKOUT:_____
Time	**Meal**	**Cal**
breakfast		
morning snack		
lunch		
afternoon snack		
dinner		
evening snack		
		TOTAL CALORIES:

TUESDAY: _____ **WATER:** _____ **WORKOUT:** _____

Time	Meal	Cal
breakfast		
morning snack		
lunch		
afternoon snack		
dinner		
evening snack		
	TOTAL CALORIES:	

WEDNESDAY: _____ **WATER:** _____ **WORKOUT:** _____

Time	Meal	Cal
breakfast		
morning snack		
lunch		
afternoon snack		
dinner		
evening snack		
	TOTAL CALORIES:	

THURSDAY: _____ **WATER:** _____ **WORKOUT:** _____

Time	Meal	Cal
breakfast		
morning snack		
lunch		
afternoon snack		
dinner		
evening snack		
	TOTAL CALORIES:	

FRIDAY: _____ WATER: _____ WORKOUT: _____		
Time	Meal	Cal
breakfast		
morning snack		
lunch		
afternoon snack		
dinner		
evening snack		
	TOTAL CALORIES:	

SATURDAY: _____ WATER: _____ WORKOUT: _____		
Time	Meal	Cal
breakfast		
morning snack		
lunch		
afternoon snack		
dinner		
evening snack		
	TOTAL CALORIES:	

SUNDAY: _____ WATER: _____ WORKOUT: _____		
Time	Meal	Cal
breakfast		
morning snack		
lunch		
afternoon snack		
dinner		
evening snack		
	TOTAL CALORIES:	

JUMP-START YOUR METABOLISM

You may work out and you may eat only nonfat food, but that doesn't mean you'll see the muscle definition and development you deserve. Your desired body is there, but it's hidden underneath a layer of subcutaneous fat. How do you get leaner and lose weight without starving yourself? The answer is to get your metabolism to start working for you. In order for that to occur, you must consider the following:

- Portion control is the most important thing when it comes to increasing your metabolism and controlling your weight. Feeling stuffed and full is not only a bad feeling, but also it means you ate too many calories. If you eat too many calories at one time, the extra calories are stored in the body and over time turn into fat. Spread you meals out so you eat five or six a day. To maximize digestion, try to make all your meals approximately the same size. You will feel satisfied, not stuffed. Your energy levels will be elevated all day long.

- You need to eat the proper combination of proteins, carbohydrates, and good fats in five or six small meals a day. The smaller portions keep you from stuffing yourself (which tends to happen when you skip meals and end up ravenous). It actually takes more energy to digest food than it does to exercise. By eating small meals throughout the day, your body is working extra hard and expending more energy just to digest your food. This, in turn, helps get your metabolism working more efficiently.

- You need to make the right choices when it comes to proteins and carbohydrates. The best proteins are, of course, fish, skinless and boneless chicken breast, lean turkey, egg whites, low- or nonfat cottage cheese, and low-sugar protein powders and protein bars. Examples of healthy complex carbohydrates are brown rice, oatmeal, wheat bread, high-fiber/low-sugar cereals, and all fruits and vegetables. A balance of around 40 percent protein, 30 percent carbohydrates, and 30 percent good fats is a good place to start. You may need to adjust this according to your activity level, age, and fitness goals. You never want to have carbohydrates by themselves; adding lean protein and a small amount of good fat slows the rate of carbohydrates being converted to sugar and helps keep insulin levels balanced throughout the day.

- Now, you can't forget about the all-important essential fatty acids oil that your body needs to help burn fat. So often, people make the mistake of eating only nonfat foods in too large portions, without realizing the enormous amount of calories they take in per day. Further, they fail to complete their diet with the essential fatty acids necessary to change their body composition and stay healthy. For example, salmon and almonds provide the omega-3 and omega-6 fatty acids that your body needs to function correctly. I take a synergistic combination of eight oils, including rice oil, soy oil, wheat germ oil, lecithin, olive oil, pumpkin seed oil, and cod liver oil, on a daily basis. As a result, my body receives a complete balance of vitamins A, D, E, F, and K. This not only helps burn fat, but it also regulates my hormonal balance and carbohydrate cravings throughout the day.

- Dehydration is definitely your enemy. On a daily basis, your goal should be to take in between 90 and 128 ounces of water. I ask that you eliminate all juices (they are concentrated sugar with very little fiber), regular and diet sodas, and sugared/flavored drinks from your diet. If you choose to consume them, do so in strict moderation. Beverages with caffeine should be limited as well, because they only serve to dehydrate you due to their diuretic effects. Drinking sufficient amounts of water will not only keep you looking healthy and feeling better, but it will also keep the hunger pangs at bay and help prevent you from unwanted "mindless" snacking.

- So many people think that the only way to lose weight is to spend hours doing "cardio" at the gym. I've talked about creating a hormonal balance in your body and controlling your insulin levels. Exercise is the key to speeding up your metabolism and keeping that balance and control. Your exercise program MUST include resistance (weight-bearing) exercises, as well as sufficient cardiovascular challenges. As a result of including weight-bearing exercises, you'll build more lean muscle mass. Lean muscle mass burns more calories at rest, which means you'll be able to maximize your weight loss.

I know that if you accept these changes as a necessary part of the Ultrafit program, you'll find the success you desire. Good luck!

KICK THE PLATEAU

"I just want to lose those last 10 pounds!" Sound familiar? It may be the reason you originally bought this book. It may be the point you're now at after following the programs in my book. Most important, it's not uncommon to reach a plateau after following a fitness and nutrition program, especially as you get closer to your target goal. If your weight-loss progress appears to have run out of gas, here are three great strategies for jump-starting it back into action.

1. Vary Your Foods

Sometimes while trying to watch fat, carbohydrate, and caloric intake, we tend to get into a food rut by eating the same things every day. Try changing your diet on a daily and weekly basis, while remaining within your nutritional program. You may find that your body reacts positively to the variety in your diet by dropping those last few dreaded pounds and inches.

2. Rev Up Your Exercise Program

A weight-loss plateau may be the result of your body getting used to your daily workouts. By changing your workouts regularly (i.e., cross-training) and intensifying them, you will keep your body from becoming complacent with your fitness efforts. If you've been following my fitness calendars and your program has stalled, you need to look at changing your intensity levels. Try wearing a heart rate monitor. This will help you learn how hard you can actually push your body within safe limitations. Remember, if you lose weight too quickly, you will lose lean muscle mass as well as body fat, so be sure to stick to a program that gives you no more than a two-pound-per-week loss, and give yourself one or two days of rest per week. Building and maintaining lean muscle mass with regular exercise helps burn calories and boosts metabolism, so rev it up!

3. Get Back to Basics

If you've noticed a plateau in your weight-loss progress for several weeks, and are getting frustrated with that pesky few pounds that seem to be hanging on for dear life, never fear—it's time to get back to basics. Take your nutritional program back to the beginning. Are you still as strict as you were when you started the program? Are you skipping meals? Are you skipping workouts? If you're no longer keeping a food and exercise journal, you need to start it right back up. Take your measurements again and take another set of pictures so that your stats are current. Be accountable for your actions and you'll see your body respond and shed those extra inches in no time at all.

BEWARE OF DIET DANGER ZONES

- **WORK:** Peer pressure, vending machines, conference room leftovers, birthday parties, and happy hours can easily sabotage you. Don't let it happen! Take the opportunity to introduce healthier food options into the office setting. Make sure you keep your own supply of healthy snacks (such as a jar of almonds or low-sugar protein bars) in your desk, and stay away from the junk food.

- **WEEKENDS AT HOME:** Boredom often leads to unnecessary snacking, which just starts to spiral downward over the course of a lazy weekend. You need to get yourself away from the kitchen and out of the house. If you want to relax, try the library or a local coffee shop. At least there you'll have to pay for the food you eat!

- **SPECIAL OCCASIONS:** I know you don't want to have to deprive yourself when you're out with friends and family, but incorporating the Ultrafit program into everyday life is your ultimate goal. You need to have a plan; it's when you are unprepared that the most damage can be done. Speak up when it comes to making restaurant decisions. Make choices ahead of time about setting limits. However you decide to approach it, a little preparation is always better than none at all.

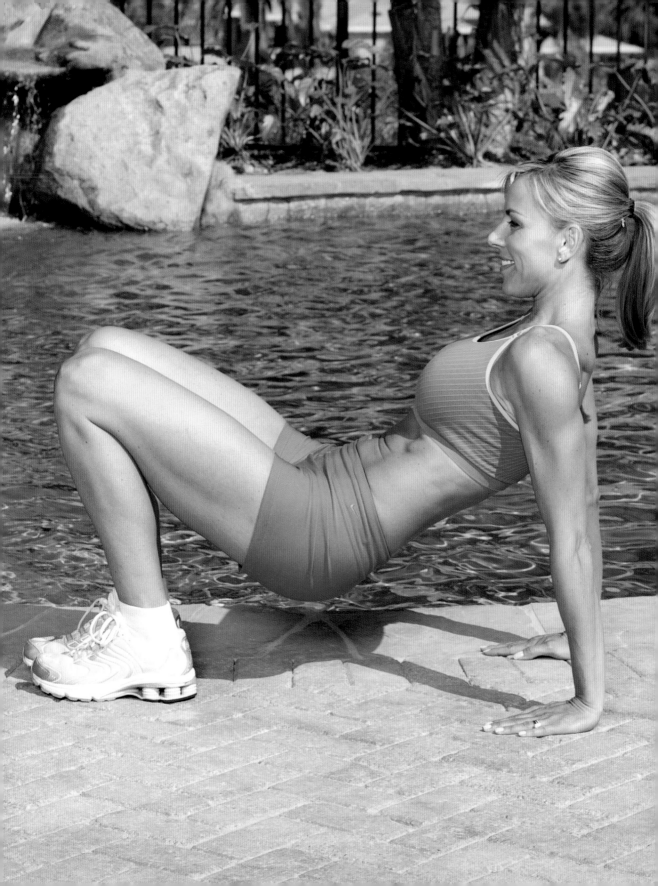

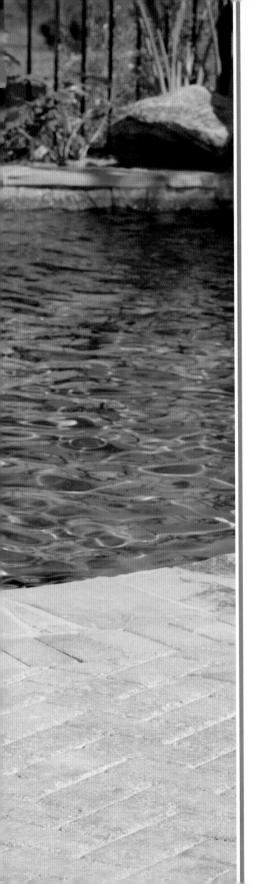

words of encouragement

It's important to remember that achieving a healthy body starts with a healthy mind. Below is an excerpt written by my friend, the famous psychologist Dr. Brian Alman, who has great advice and tips on how to achieve the mental health aspect of total Ultrafitness.

ADVICE FROM DR. BRIAN ALMAN

I think we can all agree that the best way to lose weight is to exercise more and, as you eat more intelligently, practice portion control. However, 95 percent of all diets fail because unless you change the way you think, feel, and see yourself, you will gain the weight back, and oftentimes more. Most people never discover or even consider the answers to the three most important questions they need to ask themselves if they want to lose weight and keep it off:

> *Why did you first gain weight? (What was happening in your life at that time? Why then, and not two years earlier or two years later?)*
>
> *Why did you regain the weight after losing it on a diet?*
>
> *What are the advantages to your being overweight?*

To find out the answers to these questions, you can read my book, *Keep It Off*. It will make all the valuable learning from your Ultrafit program help as much as it should. I have put together this exercise to help you start thinking positively.

Positive Self-Talk Exercise

Learning from your past successes is important, but perhaps even more important is learning to support and encourage yourself with positive self-talk.

One of the significant discoveries in psychology in recent years has been our understanding of the role our own casual self-talk plays in shaping our lives and our bodies. For example, how can you expect much success with weight loss and weight (self) management when you're continually telling yourself things like, "I'm going nowhere in my life. I just can't do this. Every time I try to change, I fail. I just don't like me. Why should I try if it's not going to work anyway? I'm no good. I'll always be fat. Just this once won't hurt. I can't help myself. I don't know what's wrong with me. I've tried but I just can't."

These are the kinds of messages we've heard about ourselves from others, messages we've heard so often that they've come to define our own self-image and direct our daily lives.

How much better you could be doing if you were saying to yourself things like, "I'm making progress with my self-care. I can handle this. I'm getting control of my weight. I am willing to try. I'm good at this. Just this once I won't. I feel more accepting and loving toward myself all the time. I feel especially good about my new skills. I'll keep trying self-hypnosis and I'll get it."

Unfortunately, very few of us have been taught how to have this sort of positive attitude about ourselves. On the contrary, from childhood we've been programmed by our parents and teachers (well intentioned, no doubt) to be negative about ourselves, to humble ourselves, and to limit ourselves, fearing that, if given our freedom, we might become too arrogant and egotistical, too assertive and outspoken and disobedient.

Eventually, we grow up and take charge of our lives, but the old programs continue to control our self-talk, our self-care, and thus our weight and body image. And so we reach adulthood overweight and gaining more weight as the years go by. Then we're faced with a dilemma: Do we settle for the body we were programmed to have, or do we try to change somehow, go back to self-care school now when we're on our own, and find our real, authentic body?

If we leave our self-care to chance, as we had to do as children, we can be certain that we'll fare no better in the future. Our bodies will be the mirror of our negative self-talk. Unless we do something for ourselves now, we're destined to live out our lives mismanaged and unsatisfied.

The decision is ours. We can manage ourselves with negative words that discourage us and lead to weight gain or with positive words that give us confidence and encourage weight loss.

Keep It Off techniques are the best way I know of to reprogram self-talk, which makes it perhaps the most powerful toolbox available for building a new positive attitude about your weight and your body. To change your attitude, or inner atmosphere, I want you to repeat any eight of the following sentences, or any ones like them, in your self-talk sessions at least once a day:

"I accept my body and I am glad that it is working as well as it is."

"I'm glad to be alive and I've decided to take the best care of my health as I can."

"Today is a really good day. I'll have other good days, but today is special."

"Today I choose to relax about my relationships and eat healthy all day."

"I can do it. Just watch me."

"I take responsibility for myself. Only I determine how I look, how I feel, the choices I make, and the decision to eat intelligently."

"I only eat foods that are good for me."

"I enjoy eating right."

"Eating a meal or a snack, I taste every bite, eat slowly, and relax in the present."

"I consistently eat like a person who weighs _____ pounds." (This should be the goal weight that you've decided on.)

"I know that how I look, what I weigh, and how I feel are 100 percent my responsibility, and each day, each night, and each moment I do everything I can to create the real me."

"I've already decided and am 100 percent committed to taking control of my self-care—and that includes how I look and what I weigh."

"I know the best way to lose weight and keep it off is to believe in myself, take control of my choices, and see myself the way I really want to be."

"I know my weight depends totally on my perspective, and I see myself as becoming lighter, healthier, and happier every day."

"Each day, before I get out of bed in the morning, I relax and become aware of my new self. I set my goals, I see myself achieving them, and I love them."

"I'm ready, willing, and able to do what it takes to feel and look the healthy way I want to. It may be difficult, but I'm worth it."

"The more I listen to my second watcher, the more I recognize the true, authentic me (inside and out)."

Give this exercise some time. Within three days to three weeks, you'll find yourself integrating positive self-talk into your life each day, all day. This will positively, absolutely, enjoyably, and naturally help you lose weight and keep it off!

Best wishes,
Dr. Brian Alman

resources and recommended reading

Aerobics and Fitness Association of America. *Fitness: Theory and Practice, Second Edition,* edited by Peg Jordan, RN. Stoughton, MA: Reebok University Press, 1997.

Alman, Brian M., PhD. *Keep It Off.* New York: Dutton Books, 2004.

American College of Sports Medicine. *ACSM Fitness Book.* Indianapolis, IN: American College of Sports Medicine, 1992.

Chu, Donald A., PhD. *Explosive Power and Strength.* Champaign, IL: Human Kinetics, 1996.

Cotton, Richard T, and Ekeroth, Christine J., eds. *Lifestyle and Weight Management: Consultant Manual.* San Diego, CA: American Council on Exercise, 1996.

Karter, Karon. *Pilates Lite.* Gloucester, MA: Fair Winds Press Publishing, 2004.

Kosich, Daniel, Phd. *Get Real.* Idea International Association of Fitness Professionals, 1995.

Kraus, Barbara. *Barbara Kraus' Calories and Carbohydrates, Fifteenth Edition.* New York: Signet, 2003.

National Strength and Conditioning Association. *Essentials of Strength Training and Conditioning,* edited by Thomas R. Baechle and Roger W. Early. Champaign, IL: Human Kinetics, 2000.

Radcliffe, James C., and Farentinos, Robert C. *High-Powered Plyometrics.* Champaign, IL: Human Kinetics, 1999.

Rinzler, Carol Ann. *Nutrition for Dummies, Third Edition.* Indianapolis, IN: Wiley Publishing, 2004.

Sheats, Cliff, and Greenwood-Robinson, Maggie. *Cliff Sheats' Lean Bodies.* New York: Warner Books, 1995.

Twining, Glenda, with Jones, Arnold Wayne. *Yoga Fights Flab.* Gloucester, MA: Fair Winds Press Publishing, 2004.

Twining, Glenda, with Seal, Mark. *Yoga Turns Back the Clock.* Gloucester, MA: Fair Winds Press Publishing, 2003.

Webb, Tamilee, with Fenton, Cheryl. *Tamilee Webb's Defy Gravity Workout.* Gloucester, MA: Fair Winds Press Publishing, 2005.

useful contact information

Cindy Whitmarsh
Ultrafit Nutrition Systems
P.O. Box 489
Solana Beach, CA 92075
www.ultrafitnutrition.com

Dr. Brian Alman
www.keep-it-off.com

Frogs Club One
www.clubone.com

IDEA Health and Fitness Association
www.ideafit.com

National Association of Sports Nutrition
www.nasnutrition.com

Nfiniti Sports, Power Reactor
www.powerreactorfitness.com

Tamilee Webb
Webb International Inc.
www.tamileewebb.com

Todd McKendrick
www.theperformancelab.net

Cindy's Clothing Sponsor: Nike
www.nike.com

Cindy's Sunglasses Sponsor: Oakley
www.oakley.com

acknowledgments

To Fair Winds Press: Thanks so much for trusting me to write a book about Ultrafitness. Thanks to Holly, Rosalind, and my favorite editor, Ed! Thanks also to Alan and Bevan.

To my Ultrafit book contributors: To Hannah Sansone for her huge contribution to this book. Your organizational skills and all the time you spent helping me make sense were invaluable! Thanks for leaving me when you had your baby! You don't need time off! Just kidding, you're the best! Second, I want to thank Dodi Benko-Livingston for her exercise descriptions, Neil Mallinson for his perfect modeling and form expertise, and Sarah Hudson for her help with the photo shoot. I couldn't have done it without you guys!

To Mike and family: My biggest thanks goes to my husband, Mike, for his constant support for me and my business. I would never be where I am in life without you! You are the greatest shipping manager and the cutest Mr. Mom. People always ask me how I handle all the projects I have going and I always give credit to Mike for being the best husband ever! Next, to my two babies, Jaden and Kendall: Thanks for letting Mommy work so much and for all the hugs and kisses when I get home! I love you! To my mom and dad, Mona and Ken, for letting me try fitness and nutrition as a career even though I knew you wanted me to go to business school. Your support my whole life has made me a confident and strong person! To the Chaussees, Vogels, Hills, and Whitmarshes: Thanks for all the support and help you give our family!

To my Ultrafit staff: First, I want to thank Trish Vasper, my Ultrafit general manager, for her tireless work and dedication to making Ultrafit Nutrition Systems so successful! To Jessica Janc, for being my first consultant and for all her creative ideas and constant dedication to Ultrafit.

Thanks to all the Ultrafit trainers for all your ideas that I love to steal! Specifically, Neil, Will, Dustin, Craig, Martin, Marney, Sandra, and all the other Frogs Club One trainers who teach for me and inspire me!

To Frogs Club One: Thanks for your awesome clubs out of which I run my Ultrafit program. Specifically, thanks to Jim Mizes, Clair Bullas, and Amy Boone for their knowledge and great business sense. Thanks to my favorite Group Ex Manager, Carrie Weiland, for always being so supportive of my career and getting me subs for all the times I am away. You are such a good friend and manager!

To Jeff Kotterman (NASN): Jeff, thanks so much for teaching me sports nutrition and for the knowledge and support you lend to all my projects, and specifically this Ultrafit book.

To Kimberly Monday and staff: Kimberly, thanks for all your amazing marketing ideas, and thanks to your staff for making my Web site and materials look so good.

To my clients: Oh, my gosh, do I love all of you!

To Hample Construction: Thanks Danny and Jackie, for allowing us to shoot the photos for this book in your beautiful home and for being such great friends!

To Anchor Bay and friends: To Michelle Rygiel, Kim Kisner, Andrea Ambandos, and Melissa McNeese, for trusting me to star in your 10-Minute Solution, Target Toning video.

To Nfiniti Sports: Thanks you for trusting me to cohost your infomercial for the amazing Power Reactor and for being like big brothers to me. Sean, Geoffrey, Tyson, Craig, and Aaron, I love working with you and I'm excited for our future!

To Nike: Thank you Eddie, Shane, and Nike, for believing in me to represent your apparel and your company!

To Oakley: Thanks, Oakley and Al for your rad sunglasses and support!

To my friends: Nikki, Cindy, Susan, Misha, Kersten, Nicole, Jessica, and Margo —you girls keep me sane. Thanks to my guy friends, Jimmy, Donny, Richard, Robert, and Danny, for keeping Mike busy for me so I can work!

To my television friends: KUSI News and Susan Lennon for giving me my start in television. Thanks to Fox 6, Desiree Carvajal, Mark Baily, and Kelli Gillespie for your support in all my endeavors.

To the people who help make me look good: Nicole Howard, Debra Phillips. To Jen Villanueva and to Shelby Ernst, for taking the North Dakota out of my hair!

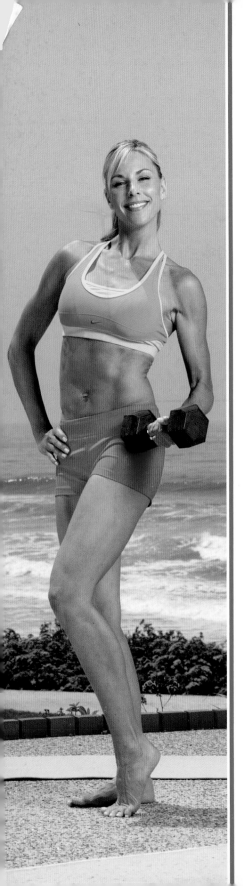

about the author

Today a celebrated nutrition and fitness guru, Cindy Whitmarsh is the owner of Ultrafit Nutrition Systems, a fitness and nutrition consulting business she runs out of four Frogs Club One Health Clubs in Southern California and is expanding throughout the state. Cindy is a licensed sports nutritionist and fitness instructor. She is the creator of the *Ultrafit Fat-Burning Workout* video and starred in the *10-Minute Solution, Target Toning* video. She is the author of *Ultrafit Cooking* and a regular contributor to numerous fitness and nutrition publications, as well as local radio and television programs. Cindy also writes nutrition and fitness programs for fitness videos, other fitness experts, and Web sites. Creator of her own annual fitness competition, The Ms. Ultrafit Competition, Cindy also co-hosts a national infomercial for Power Reactor Fitness and is the health and fitness reporter for KUSI, a television station in San Diego. Cindy also has her own radio show called *The Weight Loss Hour* co-hosted by Dr. Brian Alman.

Her high-profile clientele includes numerous television personalities, radio DJs, and professional athletes, including her husband, pro beach volleyball player, Mike Whitmarsh. Cindy and Mike have two baby girls. Cindy is passionate about health, wellness, and longevity, and she loves to share her experience and results with the world.